Praise for The Plant

"*The Plant-Based Solution* uses real-life case studies and concise explanations of science to reveal how plant-based comfort foods can bring about a vibrant, healthy life. It's compelling and well researched."

BRIAN WENDEL
president of Forks Over Knives

"*The Plant-Based Solution* is a powerful Rx for health that combines the wisdom of a doctor who spent thirty years treating life-threatening clogged heart arteries with his passion for disease prevention. He eloquently describes why even though coronary heart disease is still the number-one cause of death, it's completely preventable for most people—today. And what's good for you is also good for our planet, so healing occurs at all levels."

DEAN ORNISH, MD
founder and president of Preventive Medicine Research Institute,
author of *Dr. Dean Ornish's Program for Reversing Heart Disease*

"If you are serious about increasing both your LIFESPAN and your HEALTHSPAN, then *The Plant-Based Solution* is for you! Dig in as Dr. Kahn shares his wisdom and learnings from over thirty years as a visionary cardiologist at the forefront of treating disease with the most powerful medicine on the planet . . . plant-strong foods!"

RIP ESSELSTYN
founder of Engine 2

"Hands down, the science is irrefutable—there is no question that eating more plants makes you healthier and, as Dr. Kahn contends, "sexier" too. Knowing this information, how can anyone pass up the opportunity to eat more of these enlivening colors every day? Fortunately, Dr. Kahn will show you how to make this happen in creative ways."

DEANNA MINICH, PHD
author of *Whole Detox*

"Dr. Kahn shares his passion for healthy plant-based solutions in this energetic new book. As a plant-based chef, I am thrilled to see members of the medical community finally supporting the need for animal-free diets, and clearly demonstrating how practical, enjoyable, and rewarding a plant-based lifestyle can be. I applaud his work and look forward to the day these viewpoints are the normal. We will all be healthier, happier, and enjoy our food like never before."

MATTHEW KENNEY
founder and chief creative officer of Plantlab

"Joel Kahn is one of the great medical pioneers in helping patients actually preserve health, and not just curing sickness after the fact. *The Plant-Based Solution* belongs on the bookshelf of anyone serious about making the transition to a plant-based diet and living a longer, better life."

DAN BUETTNER
National Geographic Fellow and
New York Times bestselling author of *Blue Zones*

"The medical world is moving to acknowledge the health benefits of a vegan diet. It is rare, however, for a doctor to call for plants on the plate to benefit animals. In *The Plant-Based Solution*, Dr. Kahn raises the bar as a compassionate healer. Kindness to animals nurtures our humanity and presents another path for physicians to heal themselves and the planet. A must read."

GENE BAUR
president and cofounder of Farm Sanctuary and
author of *Living the Farm Sanctuary Life*

"Dr. Kahn elucidates keys to avoiding the ravages of the American diet in a very personal and entertaining way."

KIM ALLAN WILLIAMS, MD
professor and chief of cardiology,
Rush University Medical Center

"Few people bring to plant-based eating the expansive insights of Dr. Kahn. He is deeply concerned about people and planet alike, steeped in the relevant research and theory, and devoted to the practicalities of practice for his patients as a cardiologist, for his customers as a restaurateur, and for himself and his family. In *The Plant-Based Solution*, Dr. Kahn shares an empowering blend of conviction, expertise, experience, and understanding that leads reliably to a better medical destiny."

DAVID L. KATZ, MD
director of the Yale-Griffin Prevention Research Center,
founder of True Health Initiative

"In *The Plant-Based Solution*, Dr. Kahn utilizes an encyclopedic range of references that solidify his goal of establishing whole-food, plant-based nutrition as the foundation to eliminate chronic illness and optimize well-being."

CALDWELL B. ESSELSTYN, JR., MD
author of *Prevent and Reverse Heart Disease*

"It is rare to find the trifecta of a practicing cardiologist with decades of experience in plant-based nutrition, a book that outlines the sciences of the health advantages of this dietary pattern, and recipes packed with nutrition and taste. Put them together and *The Plant-Based Solution* is a must-read for your health and that of the planet. Bravo!"

MICHAEL GREGER, MD
founder of NutritionFacts.org, author of *How Not to Die*

"This book will change your life. *The Plant-Based Solution* gives you everything you need to put the power of food to work for health. With Dr. Kahn's medical and scientific expertise and his engagingly simple, no-nonsense approach, this book will put you on the path to success."

NEAL D. BARNARD, MD
president of Physicians Committee
for Responsible Medicine

"Dr. Kahn is a beautiful, living, breathing example of what the future of medicine will be. His practice is the perfect blend of kindness and honesty while empowering his patients with the tools to live healthier lives. *The Plant-Based Solution* is a guide to preventing chronic diseases in an affordable and delicious way that your family will enjoy and benefit from."

MARCO BORGES
author of *New York Times* bestselling *The 22-Day Revolution*

"Wow—how could anyone read *The Plant-Based Solution* and NOT want to go vegan? Dr. Kahn pulls no punches as he presents page after page of incontrovertible evidence for the astounding health benefits of a plant-based diet, in a surprisingly readable style that is infused with passion, personality, and the perspective that only comes from thirty-plus years practicing lifestyle medicine. If you're looking for all the motivation you'll ever need to change your diet, read this book."

MATT FRAZIER
plant-based ultramarathoner, author of *No Meat Athlete*

"Dr. Kahn offers the world a clearly preferable alternative to heart attacks and stent operations. This amazing cardiologist will save your heart, literally, by teaching you a simple way to prevent getting sick in the first place. Read this book. Add years to your life. It could literally save your life."

JANE VELEZ-MITCHELL
New York Times bestselling author and journalist

"*The Plant-Based Solution* is filled with passion, power, and persuasion in adopting a whole-food, plant-based diet. From rants to recipes, this book covers it all. Joel Kahn is really a Doctor of Vegetable Wisdom—I should know—he saved my life, and he can save yours too. Read this book before it's too late!"

STEVEN C. FISCHER, PHD
nutritional psychologist

"If you want to seize control of your health and the health of the planet, then this is the book for you. Born out of decades of clinical experience, Dr. Kahn guides us through the how and why of plant-based nutrition. This book is a lifesaver."

ROBERT OSTFELD, MD
director of preventive cardiology, Montefiore Health System

"Dr. Kahn describes the path of optimizing the mind, body, and spirit using compassionate nutrition focused on health, the planet, and kindness to animals. The lessons in *The Plant-Based Solution*, combined with the recipes, are a fast track to both feeling good and doing good."

JASON WACHOB
founder and CEO, mindbodygreen.com,
author of *Wellth*

"Why not reverse high blood pressure and obliterate heart attacks instead of merely managing them to reduce risk a bit? In *The Plant-Based Solution*, Dr. Kahn lays out the evidence to save millions of lives and our bloated and ineffective health-care system."

JOEL FUHRMAN, MD
president of Nutritional Research Foundation,
New York Times bestselling author

"Dr. Kahn is one of my favorite experts when it comes to healing the body from inside out. I love his approach on preventing disease through nutrition."

DONOVAN GREEN
personal trainer to Dr. Oz, founder of mygreenliving.com

THE
PLANT-BASED
SOLUTION

Also by Joel K. Kahn, MD

Dead Execs Don't Get Bonuses:
The Ultimate Guide to Surviving Your Career with a Healthy Heart

The No B.S. Diet: Science-Based Recommendations
to Stay Healthy and Medication Free Without the B.S.

The Whole Heart Solution: Halt Heart Disease Now
with the Best Alternative and Traditional Medicine

Vegan Sex: Vegans Do It Better
Coauthored with Ellen Jaffe Jones and Beverly Lynn Bennett

THE
PLANT-BASED
SOLUTION

AMERICA'S HEALTHY HEART DOC'S PLAN
TO POWER YOUR HEALTH

JOEL K. KAHN, MD

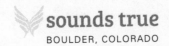
sounds true

BOULDER, COLORADO

Sounds True, Inc.
Boulder, CO 80306

This book is not intended as a substitute for the medical recommendations of physicians or other health-care providers. Rather, it is intended to offer information to help the reader cooperate with physicians and health-care providers in a mutual quest for optimal well-being. We advise readers to carefully review and understand the ideas presented and to seek the advice of a qualified professional before attempting to use them.

Some names and identifying details have been changed to protect the privacy of individuals.

Published 2018, 2020

Cover design by Rachael Murray
Book design by Beth Skelley
Cover photo © Olha Afanasieva, shutterstock.com

Kale and Sweet Potato Salad with Dried Cranberries, Kidney Bean and Lentil Dal, and Stirred-Not-Fried Wild Rice recipes were reprinted with permission from Forks Over Knives.

Cinnamon Almond Date Bites, Veggie Reuben with Cashew Cheese, Spicy Baked Potato with Broccoli and Vegan Queso, Cauliflower Purée with Sautéed Mushrooms, and Curried Gnocchi with Golden Beets recipes were reprinted with permission from VeggieChick.com.

Portions of the "Factory Farming" text in chapter 13 were reprinted with permission from Last Chance for Animals.

Printed in Canada

ISBN 978-1-68364-465-1

The Library of Congress has cataloged the hardcover edition as follows:
Names: Kahn, Joel K., author.
Title: The plant-based solution : America's healthy heart doc's plan to power your health/ Joel K. Kahn, MD, FACC.
Description: Boulder, CO : Sounds True, Inc., [2017] | Includes bibliographical references.
Identifiers: LCCN 2017021353 (print) | LCCN 2017022302 (ebook) |
  ISBN 9781622038626 (ebook) | ISBN 9781622038619 (hardcover)
Subjects: LCSH: Veganism—Health aspects. | Nutrition.
Classification: LCC RM236 (ebook) | LCC RM236 .K34 2017 (print) |
  DDC 613.2/622—dc23
LC record available at https://lccn.loc.gov/2017021353

10 9 8 7 6 5 4 3

The Plant-Based Solution is dedicated to thousands of
patients who have inspired me by their continual and
successful efforts to overcome a medical system focused on
"mopping up the mess but not turning off the sink that is
overflowing." *The Plant-Based Solution* is about turning off
the faucet that leads to preventable chronic diseases.
My patients have taught me so much over the years and
have given me a reason to show up to my clinic with a
bounce in my step and the knowledge that it is going
to be another great day of progress and healing.

No disease that can be treated by diet
should be treated by any other means.

MAIMONIDES (1135-1204)

Contents

Foreword by John Mackey, CEO, Whole Foods Market

Dr. Joel Kahn is a man with a mission and a message. His mission, like any good doctor's, is to save lives. His message? Eat plants, and lots of them. *The Plant-Based Solution* is a call, by an esteemed cardiologist, to wake up to the best science and research about health, disease, and longevity. On page after page of this highly accessible and authoritative book, Dr. Kahn presents the overwhelming evidence that a whole foods, plant-based diet is unmatched in its capacity to prevent and reverse disease, revitalize our bodies, and extend our lives.

As cofounder and CEO of Whole Foods Market, I have watched from a unique vantage point as the movement toward healthy and organic eating has gathered steam. I have been tremendously encouraged by the millions of people who are taking back their health through the remarkable power of diet. I have seen lives transformed, families saved, and communities reenergized through the power of food-based medicine. Yet America's healthy eating movement, while growing fast, is still relatively small. We are still losing the larger battle for our nation's health. We are a population beset with chronic disease, most of which is a direct result of what we put on our plates. More than a hundred million people in this country are diabetic or prediabetic. Heart disease is our number-one killer. Obesity affects 36 percent of adults and 17 percent of children and brings with it a host of ills. These chronic conditions claim millions of lives and cost all of us billions in out-of-control health-care costs.

As Dr. Kahn declares in the following pages, much of this human toll is painfully unnecessary. We already know the solution. "The word is out," he writes. "Plants heal. Plants save lives. Plants reduce medical costs. Plants prevent disease." Even much-feared chronic diseases like dementia, Alzheimer's, MS, and Parkinson's, he explains, are deeply connected to what we eat.

This is actually good news. It means that our long-term health is not merely dependent on our genetics. We have the opportunity to transform our health outcomes simply by changing what's on our plates. We need not wait for dramatic medical breakthroughs, new pharmaceuticals, or ever-better procedures. The power is our hands. But to use that power, we have to educate ourselves. Those of us who live in the developed world have an unprecedented opportunity and responsibility. We don't have to worry *if* we are going to be able to eat. Getting enough calories is no longer our primary problem. Indeed, for the first time in history, it is estimated that more people will suffer disability because of too many calories than not enough calories. Never before have we had access to the sheer variety of whole and healthy foods that are available in any grocery store. And yet, never has it been so easy to cheaply consume an endless supply of highly processed, unhealthy "food-like substances," as food writer Michael Pollan calls them, that will break down our bodies and shorten our lives. In this era of endless options, we must make conscious choices to eat well. That starts with education.

I've met Dr. Kahn, heard him speak to attentive audiences about nutrition and health, read his thoughtful writings on nutrition and heart disease, and had the pleasure of dining at his wonderful GreenSpace Café in Ferndale, Michigan, where he is a gracious host. He is an example of a new kind of physician—part medical doctor, part educator, and part health advocate. He has traversed the conventional medical world and understands that surgery and pharmaceuticals only go so far. What matters far more, especially when it comes to chronic conditions, are the simple choices we make every day of our lives—what we eat and what we don't.

Unfortunately, the question "What shall I eat?" often seems to be a subject of great confusion today. That's not accidental. Significant players in the food industry have a vested interest in keeping the general public in the dark about the best nutritional advice and keeping butter, meat, eggs, sugar, and oil at the center of our diets. It's to their advantage to make it seem like nutritional science is contradictory and confusing. That is why we must rely on trusted authorities like

Dr. Kahn who have done the research and carefully sorted through the best science. He can save you from the misleading voices that tell you it's all too complex, or it's all a matter of individual genetics, or that bacon is good for you, or whatever the latest fad diet might claim. He can help save you from the illusion of confusion that has descended over our food culture in recent years. The truth about diet and health is actually quite clear: You just need to know whom to listen to.

The food industry is powerful, but it does change. And the engines of that change are shifting cultural preferences and consumer demand. Whole Foods Market is an example of this. Forty years ago, there wasn't much of a market for organic foods. Today, organic food is a growing, thriving, multibillion-dollar market, because more and more people have voted with their hard-earned dollars to make it that way. Hopefully, in forty years, we will be able to say the same thing about a dramatic shift to whole-food, plant-based eating. And by reading this book and following its advice, you can be a pioneer of that shift today.

This change in diet will impact much more than individual health. It will also transform our society in numerous ways, as Dr. Kahn lays out. Whole-food, plant-based eating is transformative to a health-care system that is ever more burdened by the cost of chronic disease. It's incredibly beneficial to an environment that is being damaged by the heavy footprint of animal agriculture. And eating a plant-based diet, as a recent *New York Times* article pointed out, may be the number-one thing that any single person can do to ameliorate the issue of climate change. Finally, it's a compassionate choice. I have spent many years working on the ethics of eating animals, and trust me when I tell you that the killing fields of our factory farms are something future generations will look back on with disbelief.

I'm a businessman, and there's nothing I like more than a deal in which everyone wins. Whole-food, plant-based eating is truly win-win-win-win. Rarely does one simple choice have such a far-reaching impact on our own lives, the well-being of our communities, the suffering of our fellow creatures, and the health of our planet. *The Plant-Based Solution* is that important. I recommend you read it closely, put it into practice carefully, and enjoy the benefits for a very long lifetime!

Preface

Let me tell you a bit about my upbringing and an important day in my life. I was raised in a home that observed kosher dietary laws of the Jewish faith. The meat we purchased—and yes there was meat—was bought at a special kosher butcher shop. We never combined milk and meat at meals. And there were some foods, like pork and shellfish, that were never in the house, as they are always prohibited.

This experience was a blessing in many respects because it elevated food to something that required mindfulness. I learned to pause before eating to consider if the content of my plate was acceptable to my tradition. Food mindfulness is a key to appreciating the miracle of health, the power we hold to choose wisely or poorly, and in staying the course on a dietary program that is different from the norm. If you have no food rules and can eat anything made anywhere, there are literally tens of thousands of choices to consider, and it can tire you out. By some estimates, there may be over 200 decisions daily on food choices, and it can be a strain. If you grew up eating kosher as I did—or eating only vegetables, fruits, legumes, nuts, and seeds as I do now—the "decision fatigue" decreases enormously, for eggs, meat hamburgers, dairy ice cream, and BLTs are never a consideration. It is actually easier to choose from a shorter list. Think of a list with five great wines versus 500 choices. Which is easier to utilize on a daily basis when you are rushed and managing your busy life?

At age eighteen I was accepted into a combined premedical/medical program and entered the University of Michigan in Ann Arbor with my long-time girlfriend, Karen, who was accepted into the nursing school at the same university. On the first day of classes I walked into the dormitory cafeteria with Karen, and we looked around. Only the salad bar looked appealing, and it also met the kosher rules we wanted to honor, so we became vegetarians. That decision has remained in place for forty years, as well as the decision to stay together—we have been married now for over thirty-six years.

The transition from college vegetarian to vegan happened after we both read the book *Diet for a New America*, which laid out the reasons a plant-based diet was ideal for health, kindness, and the planet. Around that time, my parents began visiting the Pritikin Longevity Center in Miami, where my mother, quite an accomplished cook, learned the nuances of plant-based cooking that was also very low in salt.

My plant-based commitment was sealed when I began my medical practice in Ann Arbor as a staff cardiologist and catheterization-laboratory attending physician. I had gained advanced skills during my cardiology training in balloon angioplasty and so was off and running on July 1, 1990, my first day at a busy practice. Plants powered me. All of that lasted only three weeks because my life changed on July 21, 1990.

I was going through my mail late at night and reading the medical journals that had arrived (this was before digital editions). In a prestigious British journal called *The Lancet* was a report on patients with advanced heart disease treated with either standard therapy or a program emphasizing a plant-based diet low in fat along with walking, social support, and stress management. You will read more about this study, called the Lifestyle Heart Trial, later. I did not know of the lead author, Dean Ornish, MD, but I recognized many of the other authors as leading academic physicians admired worldwide.

The report, which looked at baseline and follow-up cardiac catheterization, my specialty, claimed that blocked heart arteries became better, or reversed in severity, during a plant-based diet and lifestyle program. This had never been reported before, and I was dumbfounded but excited. I read the report over and over and was impressed by its important and potential impact in my practice. While I did not stop performing advanced catheterization procedures that day, I did start teaching my patients that the lessons from the Lifestyle Heart Trial should be adopted in their own lives to prevent further blockages and procedures. Today, over twenty-five years later, that is my only focus: teaching the early detection, prevention, and reversal of the number-one killer of men and women in the world, heart disease, along with other serious medical challenges like adult diabetes, obesity, hypertension, autoimmune disorders, and even some cancers.

I have benefited by that early introduction to plant-based eating and have acquired a deep appreciation for the impact it has had on my relationship with planet Earth and its animal population in terms of fostering a kind and caring attitude. I have been able to maintain a stable weight, a freedom from prescription medications, legendary energy, and a passion for continued learning and teaching. But enough about me. Let's get on with the Plant-Based Solution for you and your loved ones.

Introduction

I want to say it early and I will repeat it often: there is no decision you can make that is as powerful for your health and as supported by medical research as giving up all animal foods and learning to replace them with enjoyable and healthy plant-based substitutes. That is what I want to convince you of—by taking you through body system by body system and explaining the overwhelming medical data that exists for plant-based nutrition. A plant-based diet, one that is nearly or completely free of all meats, eggs, and dairy, is the answer to preserving or regaining your optimal health. When I use the term "plant-based diet," I am referring to a vegan diet, which is based entirely on plant foods without any dairy, eggs, or meats.

My strength is my knowledge of the medical science, and admittedly I am not a chef, nor do I even run the kitchen at my home or my restaurant, GreenSpace Café, in Ferndale, Michigan. After over thirty years as a physician, forty years as a vegan, and serving tens of thousands of meals to the public, I am only writing to help you from my place of authority and experience. My oath to not harm that I took as a medical doctor is the principle you can trust as you read this book.

It can be a tough world out there if we are searching for health messages to trust and follow. Most of us are looking for something to enhance our lives, boost our energy, trim our bodies, make our skin glow, or provide a sense of purpose in a world that can be confusing and occasionally scary. While we may chase the latest fad—whether it is a new skin treatment, a style of exercise, a novel nutritional supplement, or the teachings of a charismatic speaker—we often overlook one of the most profound practices literally at our fingertips to raise our health, our purpose, and our connection to others and the fragile planet on which we live with billions of living creatures. In over three decades practicing medicine in some of the greatest medical centers anywhere, I have been struck by the immense power we have in choosing to make the 65,000 or so meals we decide upon into moments of health and purpose.

The Most Powerful Choice You Can Make

Food is powerful information for our bodies, and when combined with yoga, exercise, sound sleep, stress management, and hydration, it can reverse almost any health problem. At least three times a day, we hold the power of choosing foods to honor our miraculous bodies, to promote our inner and outer health, to honor planet Earth—which is being increasingly impacted by a fast-growing population that will reach 10 billion people within our lifetime—and to honor and respect animals with a kind heart and soul rather than with a cruel and insensitive attitude. Every day can be one focused on health practices for ourselves and our loved ones. Every day we can make conscious decisions to respect the environment and make small but important steps to reduce our damage to the planet. Every meal can be viewed as an act of *ahimsa*, the Sanskrit term for non-harmfulness and compassion to ourselves and other creatures. This is the very meaning we are often searching for.

Although many different patterns of eating have sustained humans over preceding centuries, we do not live in the era of cavemen, agricultural farming societies and private farms, or lush tropical gardens. Most of us have outsourced our nutrition to big farming enterprises concentrated in the hands of a few megacorporations reporting to shareholders, to giant food manufacturers looking for shelf life and sales far beyond our biochemistry needs and planetary well-being, and to restaurants and food vendors providing us with roughly half of the meals we eat each week.

Do you know how much salt, genetically modified oils, antibiotics, hormones, and toxins might be in a meal you pick up on your way home from work? Probably not. As a restaurant owner dedicated to very high standards, I can pretty much assure you that the answer might shock you and shock your health simultaneously. But the good news is you can control the quality and content of the fuel to power your body to health or harm.

Increase Your Lifespan and Healthspan

The fact that our health is suffering physically and spiritually is without doubt. Obesity has exploded since 1985, when the Centers for Disease Control and Prevention in Atlanta began tracking and reporting an annual map of the rates of obesity in each state in the United States. Every state has seen a dramatic rise in obesity. Along with obesity follows adult diabetes; cardiovascular disease (hypertension, stroke, and heart disease); dementia; and orthopedic and joint destruction. For the first time, the fear that our lifespan may be suffering from the pressure on our health, which centers around our food chain, has been realized by a documented decrease in the average lifespan of Americans. And what about the term "healthspan"? The last ten to twenty years of a person's life is often one of progressive decline entailing the need for medications, medical procedures, and possibly facilities to provide services that can no longer be performed independently. The goal to increase lifespan and healthspan is being threatened, and we may be losing the battle.

So what can be done by every individual in the United States and in other countries? What decision can be made starting today, whether it be a sprint into making life more meaningful and healthful or a slower "inch-by-inch" approach toward the same goals? The solution is to raise a plant-based lifestyle to the center of both consciousness and dietary choices as a daily, meaningful decision to say yes to health, yes to supporting the health of our planet, and yes to kindness over the torture that characterizes the vast majority of animal-based food products consumed daily.

It is an established medical fact, one not clearly agreed upon until the last decade, that from cradle to grave, eating only plant-based foods free of all animal products (eggs, meats, dairy) can sustain and promote health at all ages. It may be necessary to take a small amount of vitamins like B12 and D to insure proper health and growth, but a trip to a farmers market, garden, or produce department can without question result in healthy babies, healthy children and teens, and healthy adults of all ages. There is no known medical reason why everyone could not thrive on a well-balanced and well-planned plant-based diet.

Furthermore, as you will see, not only is it now agreed upon that all can thrive on whole-food, plant-based (WFPB) diets alone—vegetables, fruits, legumes, nuts, and seeds only, the Plant-Based Solution—but the medical database overwhelmingly agrees that we can prevent the chronic diseases that can shorten both our lifespan and healthspan when we choose a plant-based solution daily. Even more startling is that medical conditions present for decades, such as blocked arteries, adult diabetes, obesity, hypertension, and cholesterol elevations, can respond in weeks to months when animal-based diets are eliminated and plant-based diets are chosen. This is nothing short of a plant-based miracle. You may want to take part in this miracle in your own life, whether you do it privately, share it with your family, or turn it into the central defining piece of your life's purpose as many of my friends and I have done.

I will present to you in as simple a manner as possible the reasons why the biggest health challenges we face can be lessened, avoided, or reversed by eating only plant foods. This book includes the most compelling pieces of medical research to demonstrate the scientific support for the miracle of a plant-based solution. In addition to the science, I will ask hot questions, present case studies, share tips to eat more fruits and vegetables, and go off on rants whenever needed. In the "Plant-Based Plan" boxes, I also provide suggestions for beginning your plant-based journey. In chapter 15, I provide the recipes that I love and make to impress you of the simplicity, beauty, and satisfaction you can have eating exclusively from the plant world. You will know what you need to have in your kitchen, what to buy at the store, and how to assemble enough meals to enjoy a change in palate along with the pleasure that fruits, vegetables, legumes, whole grains, nuts, seeds, and spices can provide. There are numerous online resources to help you keep learning and experimenting after you finish this book, and I list many of those in the resources section.

So hold on, stay with me to the end, and I hope you will be convinced and excited to begin the Plant-Based Solution for yourself and your family.

Plant Rant

Although I have used the word "kindness" several times in this introduction, the gloves will come off at times in this book. The case for plant-based diets is so strong that the world should have reacted to

Dr. Dean Ornish's research in 1990 and other groundbreaking pieces of research in a manner as strongly as I reacted. The recognition of the healing ability of plants should be the norm in the medical world and the world of authors and experts. Alas, there are very vocal critics and opponents who ridicule the research of Dr. Ornish and other scientists in such a loud manner that it leads to widespread confusion. Is added oil good or bad? Is butter good or bad? It can be an ugly war of sorts often played out in social media, newspaper interviews, and TV appearances. You can turn on public TV one night and view my special praising a plant-based, no-added-oil diet for advanced heart disease and adult diabetes and the next night hear the opposite message praising high levels of added fats.

Confusion was a strategy of the tobacco industry, and there is reason to believe that the egg, dairy, and meat lobbies are not far behind. This book is geared for you, not necessarily the university classrooms in which I teach. I have embraced the role of the pugilist, punching back with powerful data and case studies, and I am game for a debate when called for. Sadly, food wars and the multibillion-dollar food industry play hardball. Do not be confused. I do not accept monies from artichoke, apple, or spinach producers. This book is the product of decades of clinical experience and medical practice. Let the plant rant begin.

THE PLANT-BASED PLAN **Get Inspired**

While what you eat is something you actually can control, changing your diet is difficult. Set yourself up for success. These are the first things I ask my patients who are beginning a plant-based diet to do:

1. Watch the documentary *Forks Over Knives*. This ninety-minute film on the relationship between diet and health profiles doctors and patients and has changed thousands if not millions of lives.

2. Register for the Physicians Committee for Responsible Medicine's 21-Day Vegan Kickstart free online program. You will get a twenty-one-day meal plan, nutrition advice, and diet and lifestyle tips: pcrm.org/kickstartHome.

3. Download and read Mercy for Animals' free The Vegetarian Starter Guide, which has pointers on getting started in the kitchen and will help you appreciate the positive impact your kind plant-based diet has on animal suffering: mercyforanimals.org/files/VSG.pdf.

1

The Six Pillars of Support
for the Plant-Based Solution

The support for plant-based health is overwhelming, fantastic, amazing, fascinating, and convincing. In this chapter, I summarize the most credible scientific information that backs the health claims of the Plant-Based Solution. If you do not have the why for making changes to upgrade your health and that of the planet, you will never get to the how. So the science, even presented in a simple way, is the foundation of choosing a plant-based diet for your health over all the other options on magazine stands, bookstores, TV shows, and social media outlets.

Science can be cool and interesting and is the basis for understanding how we are alive and healthy. Admittedly, you can adopt a plant-based diet solely from either the ethical standpoint of not harming animals or the environmental view of preserving the planet. Do it! But most of you are probably reading this book because you want to feel better, regain health, reduce medications, and avoid illness. The science is necessary to show you that this is THE path you need to start and follow for as long as I have.

Over the past few decades, many people have successfully elected to eat exclusively a plant-based diet, and a large body of scientific data proves its health benefits and safety. Nonetheless, there are always naysayers and skeptics who may present opinions or experiences to the contrary: "My brother-in-law's friend's sister's boss tried to eat a vegan diet, and her cholesterol levels went to over 1,000," or "I ate plant-based for a few months and gained forty-five pounds while developing acne and gas," or so many other similar versions that can be found on the Internet. What were these people eating? Not sweet potatoes, broccoli, bean stews, and tempeh burgers or the thousands of other delicious and nutritious options available in the WFPB (whole-food, plant-based) world.

In case you run into one of these postings, podcasts, or videos that expresses the dangers of a WFPB diet, it will be important to remember the powerful but simple factors that confirm the safety and acceptability of the Plant-Based Solution for you and your family. In this chapter, I will explain these six key pillars of information that support the power of a WFPB diet. These are all *wow* moments for sure. They are strong statements for why you should begin or continue your WFPB diet starting today.

1. The 2015–2020 Dietary Guidelines

Politics, money, power, influence. These issues come into play every five years when the US Department of Agriculture (USDA) reexamines policy statements aiming to translate the latest science to help the public choose foods for a healthy and enjoyable diet. The stated goal of the Dietary Guidelines is to improve health and reduce chronic disease with the main focus on preventing diseases, like adult diabetes.

The Dietary Guidelines are often used or adopted by medical and nutritional professionals. They are also used to develop policy that impacts the USDA's National School Lunch Program and School Breakfast Program, which feed more than 30 million children each school day. The guidelines also impact the Special Supplemental Nutrition Program for Women, Infants and Children (WIC) and the Older Americans Act, totaling millions more meals daily in the United States. Finally, the Department of Veterans Affairs and the Department of Defense rely in part on the guidelines to develop food programs for the armed services and veterans. Therefore, each edition of the guidelines is a very important document developed by a panel of experts and lobbyists and then finalized and published.

For its latest Dietary Guidelines, the federal government—after many hours of meetings, presentations, and debate—chose only three patterns of eating to endorse.[1] One pattern is the Mediterranean (MED) diet, featuring large amounts of WFPB choices; the second is a US Healthy Eating Pattern, which also features many WFPB choices; and the third is a Healthy Vegetarian Eating Pattern. Of note, there is a vegan option within this third dietary pattern, the first time an all-plant-based diet received this governmental commendation.

Although vegetarian dietary patterns had been mentioned in the 2010 Dietary Guidelines, the 2015–2020 edition placed an eating pattern free of all animal products on a lofty pedestal for health promotion. This should come as some comfort when you are considering adopting the Plant-Based Solution. In the federal guidelines, soy products, legumes, nuts, seeds, and whole grains were increased while meat, poultry, and seafood were eliminated. A vegan pattern was described using plant-based dairy substitutes, like soy and other milks. The guideline indicated that this vegan option within the Vegetarian Healthy Eating Pattern was higher in calcium and fiber than other choices, although vitamin D (and vitamin B12) may be somewhat reduced and need supplementation, which is hardly a big deal.

The reaction to the vegan Dietary Guideline by plant-based medical groups was enthusiastic. Whether more plant-based options will appear in schools, federal hospitals, and childhood WIC programs is uncertain but hopeful. You can use the power of this Dietary Guideline endorsement of plant-based diets at the highest level to support your journey and fend off the trolls who will often try to knock you down (sadly, often your closest friends and family).

2. The Academy of Nutrition and Dietetics

The Academy of Nutrition and Dietetics is the world's largest organization of food and nutrition professionals and has over 100,000 practitioners. These include registered dieticians, dietetic technicians, and other professionals and students. Members are involved in health-care systems, food service, research, and private practice. They are also leaders in following and influencing dietary policy, including the federal Dietary Guidelines.

The academy presented its position paper on vegetarian diets, and it is extremely favorable. The academy's overall position states that "appropriately planned vegetarian, including vegan, diets are healthful, nutritionally adequate, and may provide health benefits in the prevention and treatment of certain diseases." These diets, according to the paper, are appropriate for all stages of the life cycle, including pregnancy, lactation, infancy, childhood, adolescence, older adulthood, and for athletes. In fact, the paper recommends starting a WFPB diet a year before getting pregnant to rid the body of mercury, PCBs, and other toxins found in animal foods.[2]

The report explains that "plant-based diets are more environmentally sustainable than diets rich in animal products because they use fewer natural resources and are associated with much less environmental damage." The paper goes on to comment that "vegetarian diets can provide protection against many chronic diseases such as heart disease, type 2 diabetes, obesity, and some cancers," as I will discuss later.[3] Wow. There is not much more that needs to be said to support your journey to follow the Plant-Based Solution. This document by the academy is a welcome summary of research and focus on the environment and of the consequences of our food choices.

3. The US Government: Medicare and Medicaid

The US government and its systems pay millions of dollars annually to doctors and hospitals. This is a big deal for understanding how powerful the support is for the Plant-Based Solution. Just follow the money. All requests for reimbursement for Medicare and Medicaid services are evaluated to determine whether they are appropriate for payment by the Centers for Medicare & Medicaid Services (CMS), an office of the federal government, only after exhaustive consideration. The CMS has approved only two reimbursable programs for intensive cardiac rehabilitation (ICR).[4] One is called the Pritikin ICR program, and the other is the Ornish ICR program. Both are plant-based programs combined with exercise and support for cardiac patients. When you hear about a new diet fad, like the low-carb, high-fat diet (LCHF) or a grass-fed meat diet, knowing that the CMS carefully evaluated and gave the stamp of approval to only two plant-based programs should serve as a reminder that you are on the right path. Wow for sure!

4. U.S. News & World Report

You might think the media was entirely in love with the Paleo diet, the MED diet, or perhaps some other recent diet fad. Actually, there are some responsible and respected media outlets that love the Plant-Based Solution. The next resource that will strengthen your conviction to embark on and maintain the Plant-Based Solution comes from a popular news and information website, the *U.S. News & World Report*.[5]

For many years, a panel of nutrition experts has ranked various diets for health. For the seventh year in a row, the best diet for heart health selected was the Ornish diet, an eating pattern based on decades of research, which you will learn more about in the next chapter. The media site also indicates that the Ornish diet can be "tailored to losing weight, preventing or reversing diabetes and heart disease, lowering blood pressure and cholesterol, and preventing and treating prostate or breast cancer."[6] That is an amazing list of benefits for a dietary pattern that was also endorsed by the CMS.

Where were the Atkins and Paleo diets, which eliminate carbohydrates and emphasize calories from fats and animal products? They were at the bottom of the list. No one in the Paleo movement mentions the *U.S. News* list, of course, but you have my permission to do so.

5. (Some) Hospitals Love Plant-Based Diets

Not all hospitals love plant-based diets, but one big and powerful system does, and you should know about it. Actually, it is rare to see medical centers act as the leaders in the movement to incorporate a plant-based diet to prevent and reverse chronic medical conditions. While it might be bad for "hospital business" if the number of cases of heart disease, adult diabetes, hypertension, and similar maladies dropped from the adoption of WFPB diets, hospital systems should see beyond the empty hospital beds to serve the public. One exception to these blinders is one of the largest not-for-profit health plans in the world, Kaiser Permanente, covering around 11 million members. In a true spirit of aligning the evidence-based health messages of plant-based nutrition with the well-being of its members, Kaiser published both a medical article describing the health benefits of a WFPB diet and also a guide for patients to get started.[7] These materials are available in offices staffed by over 17,000 physicians in the Kaiser system. Kaiser has asked its physicians to recommend a plant-based diet to *all* of their patients by encouraging WFPB eating patterns while discouraging dairy, meats, and eggs as well as processed foods. This represents a great example for all medical centers and a strong vote of support for your journey on the Plant-Based Solution.

6. Fruits and Vegetables Save Millions of Lives

If this final pillar of information that supports the power of a WFPB diet scares you, then eating a single serving of fruit or vegetables might be your goal right now. But let's dream big early. What would happen to your health if you could adopt a habit of eating ten servings of fruit and vegetables a day? This may strike you as impossible, but using a personal blender in the morning packed with produce can provide five to seven servings before you leave the house, so do not give up yet!

An international group of researchers pooled ninety-five studies involving almost 2 million study subjects who had provided dietary information on fruit and vegetable intake.[8] They looked at the risk of heart disease, cancer, and overall survival in the follow-up based on how many servings a day were consumed on average. The researchers found that eating 800 grams a day of fruit and vegetables—or about 1¾ pounds, which would be about ten servings—led to a 24 percent drop in heart disease, a 33 percent drop in stroke, 14 percent drop in cancer, and an impressive 31 percent drop in overall death rates during the study periods. They estimated that up to 8 million people a year would avoid death worldwide if they adopted the ten-servings-a-day habit.

Plant Rant

You might walk into a hospital or school cafeteria and think there was controversy over the role of a plant-based diet for health. Viewing burgers, hot dogs, bacon, pepperoni pizza, and beef chili would make it appear that a diet high in animal products, including processed meats, was healthy. I could take you into the doctors' dining room of every hospital I am on staff at and show you egg sausage sandwiches, bacon strips, and cheesy eggs. However, as I have indicated, the word is out: Plants heal. Plants save lives. Plants reduce medical costs. Plants prevent disease. I promise you that I will not stop exposing and writing about the hypocrisy that exists in medical institutions and other teaching and healing centers, including schools, until healthy whole-food, plant-based options are available or exclusive choices.

THE PLANT-BASED PLAN   **Find Support**

> If you want to walk fast, walk alone.
> If you want to walk far, walk together.
> **AFRICAN PROVERB**

Join or create a support network by finding people online or in person who follow a plant-based diet. There are nutrition support groups like the ones we have in Michigan. There are social groups and clubs that host potlucks and gatherings at plant-friendly restaurants. Search for them online or on Meetup.com and Facebook.

If you are single, you might be interested in Veg Speed Date, a speed-dating organization that hosts events across North America.

See if there is a vegetarian or vegan festival near you. These events take place around the globe to promote veganism or vegetarianism and usually offer educational lectures and foods to taste or purchase.

2

The Heart of the Matter

had a heart murmur as a child and underwent a heart catheterization when I was a year old. I do not remember that event, but I do have a good photo of my pediatric cardiologist standing at my crib and holding me and a cigarette simultaneously. I imagine that my curiosity about those visits, coupled with the fact that my murmur resolved, led me right into the area of health and wellness. The case for plant-based diets preventing and reversing heart disease is without a doubt the strongest compared to any other diets claiming to modify chronic diseases worldwide.

Simply put, the litmus test for deciding if you should follow the latest Hollywood diet is to ask, "Is there evidence that it can reverse years of heart artery damage; reduce heart symptoms; and reduce events like hospital admissions, heart attacks, bypass surgery, and stents?" If the answer is no or more likely "It has never been studied," then politely say, "Thank you, but I would rather stick with the only dietary plan ever shown to actually reverse the number-one killer I may face or am facing now." Do not be confused. There is no evidence any diet other than a plant-based one can prevent and reverse heart disease, which has left people as young as those in their thirties weakened, limited, or prematurely dead. It is the dietary pattern you want to learn about and adopt as soon as possible for your health goals.

I cannot count the number of times my patients have said, "I wish I had made better decisions so as not to have suffered this heart attack and this bypass operation." Rest assured, you will not say that if you pay attention now. Let me repeat: there is no more effective way to prevent and reverse heart disease than eating a plant-based diet naturally low in oils, sugar, and salt (along with the cessation of smoking, of course), and there is no evidence that any other diet can achieve the same outcome for your health. None. *Nada. Nunca.* Never. I think you get it. Let's turn to a case study before biting into some history and data.

Bypass the Bypass with Broccoli

I met Paul over coffee and was immediately spellbound by his story. He had developed classic angina chest pain (indicating blocked heart arteries), which first surfaced after a tennis match. Like millions of other guys and gals in their mid-fifties, he ate a typical American diet, carried extra weight, and had elevated cholesterol. A heart angiogram was performed, where a tube was passed from an artery in his wrist to his heart, and dye was injected (the same procedure I had at age one and that I have performed thousands and thousands of times on others). The results showed one heart artery totally blocked and the two others about 65 percent narrowed.

Paul's medical team surprised him by recommending a heart bypass operation, rather big news for a man playing tennis a few weeks earlier. A bypass is where a surgeon saws the breastbone open, stops the heart with a high-potassium iced solution, and sews veins taken out of the legs and arteries into the heart to literally "bypass" the blockages. I imagine it might be harder to recommend the operation to patients if it were called a detour, not a bypass. In Paul's case, he researched the problem and decided to arrange his detour operation at the world-famous Cleveland Clinic, where more detours are performed than at any other center in the world.

The night before the surgery, Paul pulled a metaphorical lucky lotto ticket. The cardiologist assigned to his case inquired if he would like to consult with a clinic physician who taught nutrition—actually a surgeon with a reborn interest in reversing heart disease—rather than undergo the heart operation. This was the first time the cardiologist had ever brought this up with a patient, but Paul was the right recipient.

Thinking of that saw about to buzz open his chest the next morning, Paul said yes to the nonsurgical alternative and checked himself out of the clinic to have a phone call with Caldwell Esselstyn, MD. Dr. Esselstyn outlined a nutritional program proven to halt and reverse heart blockages without surgery. Once he had marching orders, Paul emptied out his cupboards, refrigerator, and freezer of all animal products as well as all items made with added oils of any kind. He reformed his diet to a whole-food, plant-based diet without added oil, salt, or sugar. He learned to enjoy oatmeal every morning, a huge salad with lemon or vinegar every lunch, and a variety of other plant-based pastas and dishes at dinner. Within a few weeks Paul stopped having angina pain, began to lose his midsection bulge, and was told by his local doctor that his blood pressure and cholesterol were dropping into healthy and low ranges. To the amazement of his medical team, his repeat stress tests no longer showed signs of inadequate blood supply to the heart. It was a year after starting the plant diet that Paul first contacted me.

Today, over four years later, Paul still has not had the detour surgery or a coronary stent (a stainless steel scaffold placed in an artery to reduce blockages), and he can exercise without symptoms. No other dietary or lifestyle choice could possibly have resulted in the same improvement, a truly miraculous one. But Paul was not done with his renewed focus on health. When he called me years ago to meet for coffee, his request was to assist him in forming a support group for others following the same diet, something that had not been done locally or elsewhere around the country. After meeting for coffee I agreed, and we subsequently arranged a small hospital conference room with a modest article in a local paper and word-of-mouth advertising. Expecting twenty respondents, Paul and I were overwhelmed when over 120 people showed up for that first meeting of the Plant Based Nutrition Support Group (PBNSG, pbnsg.org). We grabbed email addresses, I gave a talk on why added oils may be harmful for heart artery function, and we planned another meeting a month later to see if the response was genuine. Indeed, that second meeting drew over 150 attendees, and we have been meeting monthly ever since.

We outgrew the hospital room and moved to a local high school with an auditorium that could handle up to 900 guests—we have filled even that huge room at times. There are now over 4,000 members of

PBNSG; a medical student division that is introducing a plant-based curriculum into several medical schools locally; dozens of restaurants offering "plant perfect," no-added-oil menus, including my own GreenSpace Café; and a list of guest lecturers rivaling what any university or conference planner could offer.

The Plant-Based Solution has worked out spectacularly for Paul and his lovely family. His energy is high, his stomach is flat, and his life has been imbued with a passion for helping others. The detour he took was from patient to counselor to inspiring thousands as he lectures locally and around the country. Thank you, Paul, a hero and success story without parallel, one that could not have occurred with any other dietary or lifestyle change.

Convinced yet? I recommend if you ever are confused by a headline touting butter, cheese, meat, or oils, ask yourself, "What would Paul do?" The Plant-Based Solution is the real deal, and you can have the same health benefits that Paul enjoys. ■

Science Corner: The Extraordinary History of Plant-Based Diets for Health

Pretend this is a novel with colorful characters who yelled at their patients, were inspired by yogis, started as dairy farmers, and changed the medical world without medical degrees. All of those characters and more are part of the history of the Plant-Based Solution. The stories of how we learned that plant-based diets are preventive and therapeutic in dealing with the number-one killer of men and women is so colorful and rich that I am going to take a deep dive into the details and share some of them with you. I think you will enjoy these background stories that explain why you would want to stop eating animals and should start eating plants and more plants.

THE INCREDIBLE TALE OF WALTER KEMPNER, MD

A remarkable nutrition experiment was launched in 1939 by a German-Jewish refugee of the Nazi regime, Walter Kempner, MD. He fed his patients rice, sugar, fruit, and a few scraps of protein. You read that correctly. What an unpopular diet that would be in today's sugar-phobic world! Sugar is painted as the sole enemy of health by some current health writers, and I would advise you to cut back on added sugars. But Dr. Kempner had other ideas. He emigrated from Germany to join the faculty at Duke Hospital at the relatively small and unknown Duke Medical School (renamed Duke University Medical Center in 1957) in Durham, North Carolina. He had a strong biochemistry background.

At that time, there was no therapy for high blood pressure, which was taking an enormous toll on many, including President Franklin Delano Roosevelt. From his science research, Kempner developed a diet that was extremely low in salt and protein, as well as added fats and oils. It was also very low in taste and palatability. Kempner was known for being rather forceful with the patients who traveled to Duke while they worked on reversing their high blood pressure, kidney failure, and hypertensive eye and heart disease. He reportedly would yell at them if they complained about the drab diet, and there are even cases where he may have whipped them (hopefully gently).

Kempner was very careful in documenting and then publishing the outcomes of his patients. The results were amazing examples of reversal of life-threatening maladies, and Kempner's work led to the famous Duke Rice Diet, as it came to be known.[1] The word got out, and ultimately thousands of people traveled from all over the world to Duke for the therapy that was nearly or completely plant-based, low in oil, and highly effective. Celebrities like Shelley Winters, Buddy Hackett, and Lorne Greene were famous guests. In the process, Duke University Medical Center grew to become the world leader that it is. Although few prescribe the Duke Rice Diet anymore, it still exists as the Rice House Healthcare Program.

LESTER MORRISON, MD: THE LA CONTRIBUTION

Let's shift the setting to Los Angeles and the clinic of Lester Morrison, MD. This internal medicine specialist was caring for heart patients and survivors of heart attacks in the 1940s at a time when such therapies were nearly nonexistent. Morrison was aware of a unique report from Norway following the end of World War II. Despite expectations that the stress of World War II might lead to a spike in heart attacks in Nazi-occupied countries like Norway, the data released after the war showed the opposite. The rate of heart attacks and cardiac deaths actually plummeted. What a surprise.

Morrison and others hypothesized that the seizure of farm animals and dairy products in countries like Norway to provide food for Germany left the population relying on largely plant-based sources. Morrison designed a dietary plan for his heart patients that emphasized omitting rich foods like cream, butter, full-fat dairy, olives, nuts, avocados, oils, glandular organs, and egg yolks. He tracked his patients who followed this diet and compared them to patients who did not alter their diet. His results were published in a well-respected medical journal in 1951, and the follow-up showed a more than 50 percent drop in deaths at eight years and an even greater decrease in the low-fat-diet group at twelve years.[2] Morrison and his pioneering work set the stage for future pioneers who confirmed his observations.

NATHAN PRITIKIN: THE FOODIE AEROSPACE ENGINEER

Why would you ever need a medical degree to change the world? Nathan Pritikin didn't have one, and he was one of the most interesting pioneers in the field of plant-based therapy for heart disease. His legacy lives on internationally, and his work can help you live a healthy life.

Pritikin was an aerospace engineer and held many patents in that field for innovations with aviation. He had a manufacturing business in Santa Barbara, California. He had an inquisitive mind and had heard of the nutrition work being done by Lester Morrison. Pritikin visited Dr. Morrison in the 1950s when he was in his early forties. He learned that his cholesterol was over 300 due to his diet rich in animal products and full-fat dairy. He performed an exercise stress test and learned that he had failed it, showing signs of advanced heart disease with a limited prognosis.

Not one to be kept down, Pritikin dug into the books and designed a plant-based regimen rich in beans and low in fat, and he combined it with walking. He lowered his cholesterol by nearly 200 points at a time when there were no drug therapies, and slowly his stress test returned to normal. Convinced the diet would work for others, he began counseling those with heart disease, obesity, hypertension, and adult diabetes and observed stunning examples of reversal.

Despite serious resistance from the medical community, Pritikin accumulated careful data and presented it at medical meetings.[3] The mainstream academic world scoffed, but the case examples were amazing. He wrote a book, *The Pritikin Diet*, which became an international bestseller and earned him an invite to be interviewed on *60 Minutes*. In one of the most popular *60 Minutes* segments of all time, Pritikin rocketed to superstar status, and the calls for help were nonstop. He opened the Pritikin Center in Santa Monica, California, and continued to record data on outcomes of guests who stayed one to three weeks.

Prior to his death in the 1980s of leukemia, he specified that he wanted an autopsy after he passed. It demonstrated clean heart arteries. The autopsy report was published in *The New England Journal of Medicine* to prove his point on heart disease reversal. His legacy remains strong after his death, and his center has moved to Miami, Florida, where it is known as the Pritikin Longevity Center + Spa. After the Pritikin program was approved by Medicare for reimbursement after a cardiac event, centers with Pritikin IRC (intensive cardiac rehabilitation) programs have flourished around the United States.

HOW DEAN ORNISH, DOCTOR AND YOGI, PROVED THE POINT

Dean Ornish, MD, is one of the most respected researchers in the field of preventive medicine. Raised in Dallas, Texas, in a comfortable family with a father practicing dentistry, Dr. Ornish was introduced early in life to Eastern philosophy when his parents invited Swami Satchidananda, an Indian religious and yoga teacher, to their home. The swami may not be a household name now, but at the Woodstock

Festival in 1969 it was Satchidananda who offered the opening words. Ornish was impressed by Satchidananda's words and yogic practice, and the two remained in contact while Ornish pursued medical training at Harvard and the University of California, San Francisco.

Ornish took a year off from medical school to design and carry out a lifestyle trial with patients with very advanced and symptomatic heart disease. The early results were astounding. Removing animal products and oil and replacing them with WFPB foods and adding stress management, social support, and walking resulted in a 91 percent reduction in angina attacks in less than a month, along with improvements in stress-test measurements of coronary blood flow.[4]

Ornish pursued additional funding and launched the Lifestyle Heart Trial with a randomization between lifestyle therapy and a control group along with advanced heart imaging using state-of-the-art PET scans and heart catheterization analyzed by computer technology. Those results, the ones that I read on July 21, 1990, stunned the world.[5] Not only could angina attacks be reduced by over 90 percent by eating a WFPB diet and incorporating the other lifestyle measures, but measures of blood flow and heart artery blockage severity improved substantially in only a year. This demonstrated for the first time that years of heart artery plaque could be reversed by lifestyle measures emphasizing a WFPB diet. The conclusion was radical and paradigm changing, and it remains a game changer today too.

Any diet that proposes to benefit health must be judged against the Ornish Lifestyle Heart Program. Ornish pursued five-year data on the study group, including catheterization data showing an even more dramatic reversal of plaque in the treatment group. Meanwhile, the control group got increasingly worse despite conventional cardiology care and follow-up.[6] Not only did blood flow improve in the Lifestyle group without further reductions in heart blockages, but hospital admissions, heart attacks, and the need for heart procedures dropped by almost 50 percent. That translated to enormous savings in medical expenses. Many of us thought that the concept of nutritional cardiology and lifestyle medicine would be recognized for the breakthrough that it was and change our practices dramatically.

In reality, Ornish was celebrated to some degree, yet to this day many cardiologists are not able to identify his research or understand its implications for benefiting patients without surgery or stenting. Although it took additional years to gather adequate numbers of patients and their outcomes, ultimately the Centers for Medicare & Medicaid Services approved the Ornish program for IRC at the same time as the Pritikin program in 2010.

There are dozens of these programs around the United States benefiting thousands of patients. I will tell you more about Dean Ornish in the next section and in future chapters. For now, know that his work is finally being celebrated by current generations of physicians for the courage, vision, and persistence to prove that heart disease is a food-borne illness that can be tamed with low-cost lifestyle measures centering on WFPB diets, stress management, and abundant love for oneself and others.

Study In-Depth: Lifestyle Heart Trial

A few studies have been so important in the treatment of heart artery disease that a focus on the research is worthwhile and deserved. The Lifestyle Heart Trial led by Dr. Dean Ornish was published in 1990, but the study continued, and five-year results described in this section were published in 1998.[7] All the participants were heart patients with blocked arteries, and some were quite sick.

One group was told to follow their own doctors' recommendations, but the other group followed a comprehensive program designed by Dr. Ornish. That group was asked to not smoke; to walk; to manage stress by breathing, yoga, and meditation; to meet regularly for support; and finally, to eat a diet of plants without meats.

Angiography, also called cardiac catheterization, is a common way to assess whether heart arteries are clean or clogged. In the lifestyle study, angiography was performed, and the degree of blockage in the arteries was measured by the most sophisticated computer systems available to insure accuracy and objectivity. In the group following the Ornish program, the average amount of narrowing decreased by 10 percent after five years compared to the baseline. This means that the arteries were open wider. In stark contrast, the control group had an increase in the average degree of blockage of 28 percent, indicating arteries that were much more blocked over the five years. Because even small improvements or worsening in arteries can lead to major changes in blood flow, the changes were accompanied by quite different clinical outcomes. The control group, those not following the Ornish program, suffered 2.5 times the number of adverse events (hospitalizations, bypass surgeries, angioplasties, and heart attacks).

I have a graph from this 1998 study hanging in my office that I point out to every patient so they can see the potential for heart artery disease reversal with lifestyle changes. The differences at five years in the degree of narrowing are impressive and meaningful. The heart benefits of adopting a plant-based diet low in fat for disease reversal should be offered to every heart patient upon diagnosis.

CALDWELL ESSELSTYN, MD: THE GOLD MEDALIST MEETS THE HEART SURGEON

I had the pleasure of meeting Dr. Caldwell Esselstyn nearly twenty years ago when we both spoke at a local Detroit plant-based conference held in an elementary school with a crowd of a few hundred. That same conference now draws over 6,000 attendants in a large convention center (vegmichigan.org).

Dr. Esselstyn, or Essy, as many call him, is a man of great integrity, passion, curiosity, and accomplishment. After he won a gold medal in the Olympics in the 1950s, he went on to marry the energetic granddaughter of the founder of the Cleveland Clinic, Ann Crile. He served in Vietnam. He had a successful surgical career focusing on breast disease until renovations in the surgical locker room paired him up with Dr. René Favaloro, the first cardiac surgeon to perform bypass surgery, the detour operation. Esselstyn's passion to learn led to his immersion in reading about heart disease. He read about cultures that had no measurable problem with the number-one killer in the Western world. He was aware of the data from Norway and the drop in heart attacks during World War II that also impressed Dr. Lester Morrison decades earlier.

Essy did not feel constrained by his training as a breast surgeon and approached the cardiology and cardiac surgery divisions at the clinic in the early 1980s, asking them to refer patients not suitable for bypass or angioplasty for a nutritional program. Along with his wife, Ann, he began studying and documenting the course of advanced heart disease patients who were encouraged to eat a plant-based diet without any added oils, nuts, or avocados. The goal was a percentage of calories from fat of about 10 percent. The data he accumulated, which was published in peer-reviewed cardiology journals, showed improved symptoms, improved sexual function, improved stress-test results, fewer hospital visits, and ultimately examples of angiographic regression of coronary lesions. Essy recently published an updated sample of nearly 200 patients and identified a high compliance rate with his program and a low cardiac event rate.[8]

In short, plant-based diets without added oils appeared to quickly heal the lining of arteries, known as the endothelium. As a side note, the Cleveland Clinic is also on a mission to be the leading example of a healthy role model for hospitals. Last year it booted out a McDonald's in the lobby that was a blight on its otherwise fine reputation. A Middle Eastern café with many plant-based options recently replaced the McDonald's. The clinic is also the first major medical system to heed the findings of the World Health Organization's classification of processed red meats, such as bacon, pepperoni, and hot dogs, as Group 1 carcinogens (substances proved to cause cancer in humans). The clinic banned these foods this year against what must have been considerable pushback from staff, guests, and even staff physicians. Dr. Esselstyn and his wife have published several successful books and cookbooks to make their program easier to follow.

Although the Esselstyns' program is considered extreme or "radical" by some, as Essy points out, sawing the chest open, taking veins out of legs, and rerouting them as temporary detours to the heart is both extreme and radical. Eating large salads, casseroles, stews, soups, and side dishes is hardly radical. Of final note, the Esselstyns have been assisted on their mission to heal by their children. Jane is a nurse who joins her parents in many cooking demonstrations. Their son Rip is a triathlete and served as a fireman in Austin, Texas. He tested his father's diet on his fellow firemen in the engine house and identified major improvements in their blood pressure, blood cholesterol, and weight in only twenty-eight days. This experiment prompted several books and the Engine 2 food line to support the Esselstyns' lifestyle plan consisting of a plant-based diet without added oils, nuts, or avocados.

JOEL FUHRMAN, MD: ANOTHER ATHLETE AND NUTRITION LEADER

Dr. Joel Fuhrman, a family physician in New Jersey, was a high-ranking figure skater in his late teens. He had a passion for nutrition early in his career and developed the concept of a nutrient-dense, plant-rich program encapsulated in his book *Eat to Live*. Dr. Fuhrman has had many successful public TV programs discussing the benefits of a nutrient-dense and plant-rich diet for weight management, diabetes, immune function, and heart disease.

In his recent peer-reviewed publication, Fuhrman reported sustained drops in body weight, cholesterol, and blood pressure in hundreds of patients following his program.[9] He included case studies of cardiac patients realizing important improvements in symptom reduction and other measured outcomes. The reports were quite convincing.

Fuhrman differed in his approach from the early work of Pritikin, Ornish, and Esselstyn by including nuts, seeds, and avocados in his patients' diets. Therefore, his diets were higher in fat than the programs taught by the others. His program does stay away from added oils. With the growing recognition that a small handful of nuts daily is associated with important reductions in a variety of maladies, including cardiovascular disease, nuts are now incorporated in small amounts into the programs of Drs. Ornish and Esselstyn. What about avocados? There is still a split jury for patients working on the reversal of serious problems like heart disease, adult diabetes, and excess weight due to the high fat content of avocados.

Hot Question: Aren't Oils Healthy?

Olive oil has become a universal sign of fine dining, as well as a touted component of the Mediterranean diet. Cooking shows, magazine articles, cookbooks, and the like constantly extol the benefits of extra-virgin olive oil. Perhaps as a result of all the great press olive oil has gotten in the past forty years, the amount of fat in our diet from added oils has skyrocketed, from about ten pounds per year to over fifty pounds a year. The American Heart Association recommends that total dietary fat intake should be less than 35 percent of our daily caloric intake, and saturated fats (found mainly in animal products, such as meat, eggs, and dairy) should account for less than 7 percent of our daily calories.[10] Perhaps you've seen popular "healthy" diets recommending that 40 to 80 percent of daily calories come from fat, something that adding butter to your coffee might push you toward. Remember that in the studies demonstrating reversal of heart disease, diabetes, and obesity, the dietary fat content was around 10 percent.

The National Academy of Sciences indicates that the amount of omega-3 fatty acids we need daily is 1.1 grams for women and 1.6 grams for men.[11] This is about 2 percent of total daily calories. If you ate only green leafy vegetables all day, you'd exceed this amount. Certainly if you make it a habit to add 2 tablespoons of ground flax seeds to your oatmeal, chia pudding, or smoothie, you will have more than enough and enjoy some great fiber and nutrients. A tablespoon of ground flax seed has 1.8 grams of omega-3 and 0.4 grams of omega-6. (Unlike flax oil, ground flax maintains all the fiber of whole flax and more of the nutrients.)

Olive oil is not a rich source of the essential fats we need, and you'd have to eat almost 2,000 calories of this pure-liquid fat to meet daily omega-3 needs. Olive oil contains active chemicals called polyphenols, which reduce the harmful effects of free radicals and are good for you, but there are many better sources of this. For example, ten berries will give ten calories and zero fat and as many polyphenols as one tablespoon of olive oil, with 120 calories and 13 grams of fat. While the MED diet is healthy, it may be healthy despite the olive oil. The diet is rich in fruits, vegetables, whole grains, and wine, and it limits meat and dairy and eliminates processed foods.

Learning to prepare foods with vegetable broths, juices, wine, and vinegars can greatly reduce the added fat that is so common in our diet.

Plant-Based Intensive Cardiac Rehabilitation

Hopefully you will never need cardiac rehabilitation after a heart attack or heart bypass operation, but I want to offer a few comments on why the Plant-Based Solution is part of that therapy. Both the Pritikin and Ornish programs have received approval from Medicare for reimbursement of their plant-based therapies combined with exercise. But what does this actually mean? Cardiac rehabilitation (CR) is a program of exercise and education for patients with heart disease. It is usually performed in an outpatient hospital facility and involves monitored exercise. With an adequate diagnosis and indication, most insurance providers will pay for CR.

Both the Ornish and Pritikin intensive cardiac rehabilitation, or ICR, programs are certified by the CMS (Centers for Medicare & Medicaid Services) for patient reimbursement. Both programs are centered around a plant-based diet and involve exercise. Additionally, patients are taught cooking skills, stress management, and lifestyle habits.

It is no small matter that the only two ICR programs approved for reimbursement by the CMS are plant-based. The scientific evidence was carefully considered and approved for these two programs alone (Pritikin and Ornish). This remains powerful evidence supporting the

Plant-Based Solution and is a reason you should adopt this dietary pattern now and not wait until after a serious heart event. "Prevent not stent," as I like to say, for your health.

Science Corner: Your Endothelium and the Plant-Based Solution

One of the reasons the Plant-Based Solution works so fast and so well in heart disease requires a basic understanding about how arteries are supposed to work. Epithelium is one of the four basic types of tissues in the body (along with connective tissues, muscles, and nerves), and it lines all organs, inside and out. A specific kind of epithelium, the endothelium, lines the 50,000 miles of arteries and the 50,000 miles of veins that course through our body, a distance that would travel nearly four times around Earth, an amazing thought. The endothelium is just one cell layer thin, like wallpaper for our arteries and veins, yet it weighs as much as our liver, which is a lot.

In 1998, a Nobel Prize in medicine was awarded to researchers who discovered some of the secrets of the endothelium. Once thought to be just a barrier between blood and the walls of our arteries, the endothelium is now understood to be the key to living a long and healthy life. The cells are thin and yet very active making hormones, permitting the passage of messaging chemicals, and maintaining proper blood-vessel function. One of the most important molecules made by the endothelium is called nitric oxide, or NO, and one of the surest signs of healthy arteries is generous NO production. The converse is true of sick arteries: They do not make enough NO, and many common diseases, including diabetes mellitus and high blood pressure, reduce NO production.

Some of the main functions of a healthy endothelium include preventing inappropriate blood clotting, relaxing arteries, promoting normal blood pressure, preventing inflammation and plaques, and facilitating glucose uptake and healthy blood sugars. You need blood flow for a lot of things in life, and men definitely need blood flow for erections.

Processed foods that are high in fat quickly damage the endothelium. If you smoke, are obese, suffer high blood pressure or high cholesterol, have diabetes mellitus, or have erectile dysfunction, you likely have endothelial dysfunction (ED) and inadequate NO production. Fortunately, it is now possible to directly measure the health of the endothelium. A blood test for a molecule called ADMA is available in some clinics. The higher the ADMA level, the lower the NO production and the more ED is present. When we heal our ED, the ADMA level drops, as NO production is boosted. A device called the EndoPAT is also used to measure ED and monitor interventions to document recovery, and I use it routinely in my preventive clinic.

If you want a healthy endothelium for wellness, longevity, optimal fitness, sexual responsiveness, and heart attack and stroke prevention, there are some things you can do that are part of the Plant-Based Solution. Eating a plant-based diet will naturally help increase your intake of dietary polyphenols, nitrates, and L-arginine (see the sidebar "Foods for a Healthy Endothelium"). Maintaining a healthy weight, avoiding smoking, managing stress, and steering clear of processed and "junk" foods are important.

The endothelium can be injured rapidly, and NO production plummets if you make food choices that are part of the standard American diet. A cardiologist at the University of Maryland recruited volunteers to have two meals on separate days while a device was on their arm to monitor their endothelial function.[12] One day a low-fat breakfast was provided, and artery health for six hours was monitored and was unaffected by the meal. On the other day, the same subjects were fed an Egg McMuffin from McDonald's. Within an hour the study subjects demonstrated a drop in endothelial function, presumably due to a reduction in NO production, and this drop peaked at four hours after the meal, not returning to baseline until a full six hours after the breakfast in the yellow wrapper. This famous Egg McMuffin study is an important reminder that food matters, food is information, and food can be a therapy for your heart and arteries when you adopt the Plant-Based Solution.

Foods for a Healthy Endothelium

Try to add one or two of the following foods to your diet every day to increase nitric oxide production and support a healthy endothelium.

basil	beets
black elderberry	bok choy
capers	celery seed
chestnuts	cloves
cocoa powder	coffee
curry	dark chocolate
flaxseed meal	garlic
greens, particularly arugula	nuts, particularly pine nuts
onions	oregano (dried)
rhubarb	rosemary
sage	spearmint
spinach	star anise
strawberries	thyme
watermelon, including the rind	whole grains, like oats and wheat germ

Why You Need to Know About TMAO

There is a revolution happening right now in our understanding of the cause of heart disease, and it's a new reason to follow the Plant-Based Solution. There is a proven connection between bacteria in our gastrointestinal (GI) tract and the risk of developing clogged arteries. We've known for years that not all cases of heart disease are explained by the traditional risk factors such as smoking, elevated blood pressure, diabetes mellitus, high cholesterol, and a family history of premature heart disease. And so a few years ago researchers at the Cleveland Clinic began searching for new causes of heart disease.

The researchers looked at many potential unknown causes of heart disease but finally focused on a compound called TMAO, or trimethylamine N-oxide. This molecule, new on the scene, is produced by intestinal bacteria as a result of our dietary choices, particularly foods rich in both choline and l-carnitine, found in eggs, meat, and fish.

In the Cleveland Clinic study, the researchers showed that TMAO increased the accumulation of cholesterol in the walls of arteries, which is the beginning of plaque buildup. Further work has also shown that TMAO prevents cleaning up of cholesterol-diseased arteries, so it's a double whammy. In the studies at the Cleveland Clinic in more than 4,000 patients, the higher the blood level of TMAO, the more advanced and severe was the heart disease.

The researchers proved it was the bacteria in the GI tract that was producing TMAO because a short course of antibiotics that wiped out GI bacteria also temporarily wiped out TMAO production. Next, to determine if omnivores are predisposed to heart disease due to their dietary choices, the team recruited vegans and paid them to eat eggs or steak and measured TMAO blood levels. What happened? Nothing. Vegans have different bacteria in their GI tract. It appears that due to long-term dietary choices, the enzyme that converts these food sources to TMAO is absent, or nearly so, in vegans.

Another study showed that fish yielded the highest circulating TMAO levels.[13] The rise in TMAO was higher following fish than beef, eggs, or fruit. The rise in TMAO began only fifteen minutes after eating a meal of fish.

In terms of a remedy, so far one study of a potent probiotic failed to halt TMAO production. And while an inhibitor of TMAO production, a chemical called dimethylbutane, or DMB, has been looked at in animal studies, its safety in humans will need further study. In the meantime, skip the eggs and meat.

Plant Rant

Doctors like Dean Ornish, Caldwell Esselstyn, and many others are some of the most honorable and admired physicians on the planet, working day after day to bring natural healing methods to millions. Lifestyle medicine is now a rapidly expanding field due to their pioneering work. Was their research always perfect? No, probably not, but any study trying to change people's eating habits long term is challenging. The only programs shown to reduce heart disease, prevent heart events, and gain approval by the CMS and other insurers are WFPB diets without added oils.

Until studies of some other dietary pattern can produce decades of follow-up and similarly impressive results, critics should quiet down and give credit where credit is due. The plant-based founding fathers have rocked the world of heart disease, opening the possibility of preventing the number-one killer in the Western world. Be bold, be a warrior for the Plant-Based Solution, and teach as many as possible this amazing news.

THE PLANT-BASED PLAN Stock Your Pantry

Because many of the staples of a plant-based diet are dry goods—grains, beans, nuts, seeds, pasta, and spices—a well-stocked pantry makes preparing plant-based meals pretty convenient. Organic is preferred if the budget permits.

Whole grains: couscous, old-fashioned oats, short-grain brown rice, millet, wild rice, farro, whole-wheat dry pasta, and quinoa

Beans and legumes (seek out BPA-free linings if canned): lentils (red, green, beluga), chickpeas, black beans, firm tofu, kidney beans, cannellini beans, navy beans, black-eyed peas, split peas

Raw nuts: almonds, pecans, walnuts, cashews, Brazil nuts

Raw seeds and dried fruit: pumpkin seeds, hemp seeds, sunflower seeds, chia seeds, sesame seeds, ground flax seeds, dried tart cherries, raisins, dates

Vinegars: raw apple cider vinegar, rice vinegar, organic balsamic vinegar, organic red wine vinegar

Oils (optional): spray extra-virgin olive oil, extra-virgin olive oil, canola oil

Sweeteners: molasses, pure maple syrup, dark brown sugar, date sugar, coconut sugar

Chocolate and carob: semi-sweet chocolate chips, cacao nibs, carob powder

Additional items: nut and seed butters like raw almond butter, roasted natural peanut butter, nondairy milk free of carrageenan additives, unsweetened organic applesauce, nutritional yeast, vegetable broth, canned tomatoes and tomato sauce, jarred pasta sauce, hot sauce

Spices and herbs: allspice, basil, bay leaves, black pepper, caraway, cayenne, chili powder, cinnamon, cumin, dill, dry mustard, garlic powder, ginger, kelp granules, nutmeg, oregano, paprika, rosemary, thyme leaves, turmeric

3

The Sweet News
about Diabetes

Heart disease has been the focus of my training and clinical experience for over thirty years. However, there is no way to practice medicine—in fact, there is no way to live in the Western world—without encountering acquaintances with diabetes almost daily. Maybe you have diabetes type 1 or 2. Or prediabetes. Or maybe relatives or spouses, coworkers, friends, or advisors carry the diagnosis. Diabetes, or more properly called diabetes mellitus (from the Greek *diabainein*, "a siphon," and *mellitus*, "like honey"), is a medical problem of massive proportion. The good news is that the adult version, called type 2 diabetes, need not be the burden it is.

When I was in medical training, we separated patients with diabetes into adult diabetics and juvenile diabetics. Juvenile diabetics usually made little or no insulin due to a failure of the pancreas, and they required insulin to survive and avoid the perils of uncontrolled blood sugars. Adult diabetics were usually overweight patients who had a degree of "insulin resistance," or IR, which we will discuss more soon. The sad reality is that many teenagers now demonstrate the same type of diabetes with the same obesity-related IR as adult diabetics. In fact, the terms have shifted to type 1 (usually juvenile but also describing adults not making insulin and dependent on it for life) and type 2 (those in whom insulin may be needed but usually the body is still making some insulin, with IR the major abnormality, and often a reversible one too).

Even if you do not have diabetes, and I hope you do not, the numbers are so huge that they require a moment's focus. More than 29 million

Americans, or 9.3 percent of the population, have diabetes. What is scary is that about one in four people with diabetes do not know it, and the damage may be ongoing.[1] Although about 1.5 million Americans receive a diabetes diagnosis each year, that number would skyrocket if all the undiagnosed citizens were tested. The number of Americans considered to have type 1 diabetes is just over 1 percent of Americans (children and adults); many more have type 2. An estimated 25 percent of people over the age of sixty-five have type 2 diabetes, and the number is growing. Over 200,000 Americans under the age of twenty have a diagnosis of diabetes, and that number is growing too, particularly with type 2 diabetes and obesity.

Ready for more shocking numbers to ponder? Prediabetes is a condition where the blood sugar is consistently elevated but not to the degree to diagnose full-blown diabetes type 2. According to the Centers for Disease Control and Prevention, over 85 million Americans could be considered prediabetic—so overall, more than 100 million Americans are dealing with blood-sugar problems, knowingly or unknowingly.[2] Diabetes is the seventh leading cause of death in the United States— about 70,000 people annually—and is listed as contributing to another quarter of a million deaths. These numbers are on the low range, as death certificates do not require mentioning diabetes as a cause.

The need for the Plant-Based Solution to prevent and treat diabetes mellitus could not be greater. Patients with diabetes, particularly adults, often have several problems that may all relate to lifestyle. For example, almost three-quarters of adults with diabetes also have high blood pressure or abnormalities of cholesterol. Therefore, the rates of dying of heart conditions and related issues like stroke are at least two times higher for people with diabetes.

Blindness from diabetes is a major problem, and a third of adult diabetics have damage to the small blood vessels of the eye, a condition called retinopathy. Kidneys take a toll from diabetes too, the largest cause of kidney failure being diabetes. About a quarter million people yearly require chronic dialysis for diabetes-related damage. Finally, because of the impact of diabetes on blood vessels throughout the body but particularly of the legs and toes, 60 percent of all amputations are due to diabetic vascular damage. The total cost of diabetic care and lost work productivity in the United States may exceed $300 billion a year, a lot of money. Diabetes mellitus is now the most expensive chronic disease condition treated in the United States, even more than heart disease.[3]

CASE STUDY
Goodbye Type 2 Damn-Betes

I met Marc Ramirez at a bookstore where I was doing a book signing. Although he was incredibly kind and polite, the passion with which he shared his story was apparent right away. He grew up in Texas, one of eight children. The family moved to Chicago where Marc excelled in sports and was recruited to the University of Michigan (my alma mater) football team. He played from 1986 to 1990 (the years I was away from Ann Arbor training to be a cardiologist), and he traveled to three Rose Bowls. However, by 2002, then an overweight and sedentary executive, he was diagnosed with diabetes mellitus, type 2.

Marc was all too aware of the consequences of diabetes, as his mother died that year of complications of diabetes after suffering from vision failure, heart disease, and kidney failure. Two of Marc's siblings also had been diagnosed with type 2 diabetes. His twin brother had a heart attack, and another brother, who receives dialysis, is legally blind and had a leg amputated.

Knowing no other path, Marc took an increasingly long list of medications, including insulin, to manage his diabetes for the next nine years. By a twist of fate, his in-laws gave him a copy of *Forks Over Knives*, a documentary about plant-based nutrition with examples of patients who reversed their type 2 diabetes with diet. He was also given a book by Neal Barnard, MD, who has conducted studies on reversing diabetes with diet. Marc and his wife, Kim, immediately realized that there was an option other than the complications of diabetes that were starting to develop. They threw themselves into changing to a plant-based diet without added fats. Within two months Marc was off all medications, a miracle compared to the prior nine years. Now, more than five years later, he remains off all medications. All complications have resolved. His weight is down fifty pounds, matching his weight at high school graduation.

He shares his dramatic experience with others by lecturing and counseling people around suburban Detroit and the United States. He and his lovely wife have become certified as Food for Life nutrition instructors to help teach others the power of plants to reverse this terrible disease. Marc's Latino heritage raised his risk of developing type 2 diabetes, but his diet high in processed foods and oils pulled the trigger. Fortunately, Marc now has a bright future to enjoy with Kim and their children. He also has regained his full erectile function—which diabetes was stealing—and smiles about that now with satisfaction. Marc's story can be your story if you walk in his shoes. ■

Monitoring Diabetes

The HgbA1C blood test, also called the hemoglobin A1C or the glycosylated hemoglobin test, reflects a person's average level of blood sugar over the prior two to three months. People who have been diagnosed with diabetes have this test regularly and aim to keep their levels below 7 percent. The normal range is between 4.0 and 5.6 percent and can be achieved by many type 2 diabetics on a whole-food, plant-based, no-added-oil diet that favors weight loss and reversal of their condition. A level between 5.7 and 6.4 percent indicates significant insulin resistance and is often called prediabetes.

CASE STUDY

Fruit-Strong Diets for Type 1 Diabetes

Because diabetes type 1 and 2 are so different, the story of Robby is very important because you may have type 1 diabetes or know someone with type 1. When I first met Robby, I was impressed by his upbeat spirit. He was working as a marketing associate for Forks Over Knives, the organization that produced a documentary by the same name (that you should definitely watch), which led to books, classes, and food services.

Robby and I met over dinner, and what he ate was extraordinary. The only thing bigger than his smile was his bowl of raw veggies and fruits that he had brought along. Robby ate and talked about his journey with type 1 diabetes. He was twenty-six when we met and had been dealing with it since age twelve. Robby's treatment began with insulin and standard diets, but he was looking for something better, closer to a cure, if possible. He found an online forum discussing vegan diets for diabetes and began trying a program described by Gabriel Cousens, MD, in Arizona to cure diabetes with raw foods.

Robby lost too much weight, but this led him to another program that taught a high-carbohydrate, raw, plant-based diet called the 80/10/10 diet (a minimum of 80 percent of calories from carbohydrates and a maximum of 10 percent each from protein and fats). The diet plan centered on sweet fruits like bananas, figs, papayas, and mangos, which might shock some people, but Robby was all in. He studied the literature beginning with Dr. Walter Kempner, of the Duke Rice Diet, and another (James W. Anderson) from the 1950s reporting the reversal of type 2 diabetes in sixty-eight of eighty patients on a low-fat, high-carbohydrate diet. About 10 percent of the calories were from fat in those early research studies, and Robby patterned his diet, which he calls a fruit-based diet, after them.

Since adopting this diet, Robby has been able to maintain his diabetes with excellent control. Of course, type 1 diabetes does not go away and requires daily management. His HgbA1C has been maintained at around 6 percent with less insulin than he used to use. He notices he can manage double the calories from a raw, carbohydrate-rich diet than he once could. He eats about 720 grams of plant-based carbohydrates a day (4 calories per gram), and his average insulin needs are forty units daily, including his long-acting basal insulin. He eats three to four meals a day that add up to about 3,000 calories. Robby often has a fruit breakfast to start the day after a solid workout, a fruit meal for lunch, a fruit snack in the late afternoon, and a large salad with more fruit for dinner. He includes greens, like lettuce or arugula, with almost every fruit meal, and his salads each night include a large amount of greens and vegetables, such as lettuce, zucchini, celery, cauliflower, and others. (See chapter 12 for a discussion on daily protein requirements.)

I have had the pleasure of shopping in the farmers markets of Los Angeles with Robby, and his big smile is matched by his big knowledge of produce and the purveyors he buys from. He can name the many types of avocados, spinach, persimmons, and oranges that he enjoys. He literally loads a cart twice a week to have pounds of fresh produce at his home. Similar to Marc and Kim Ramirez, Robby has felt the calling to share what he has learned with others. Recently, he has left Forks Over Knives and has established his own diabetic counseling business along with another passionate individual with type 1 diabetes. You can find Robby and Cyrus Khambatta, PhD, at Mastering Diabetes (masteringdiabetes.org). Please be sure you discuss your diabetic program with your medical team before you make any changes. ■

Science Corner: How Do Plant-Based, Low-Fat Diets Help Diabetes?

Are you curious how you can reverse type 2 diabetes or improve type 1 diabetes with the Plant-Based Solution? A shared theme in the remarkable stories of Marc and Robby is that both men follow diets that are low in overall fats, with no added fats. There are no bottles of olive oil or sticks of butter in their homes. In fact, both shoot for about 10 percent of calories daily from fat. Robby follows the 80/10/10 formula that expressly sets 10 percent as a goal. And it works for him despite eating pounds of whole fruit daily! The usual understanding is that when you eat foods rich in sugar or refined carbohydrates, like donuts, cakes, or cookies, your blood sugar will rise rapidly. Undoubtedly, that is true, but is that the cause of diabetes, particularly type 2 diabetes, where the pancreas is still capable of making at least some insulin, or is it just a consequence of another nutrient problem?

The focus on the cause of type 2 diabetes has shifted to fat content of the diet and the ability of high-fat diets to clog up cells, making them incapable of responding to the insulin that the pancreas releases.

In fact, in a study done as far back as the 1920s, healthy people given high-fat meals or carbohydrate-rich meals had a much more rapid rise in blood sugar with the fatty foods.[4] How does this work? We store energy in our muscles, and it can be either carbohydrate-derived glycogen or fat-derived small droplets within the muscle cells. About 85 percent of the glucose in our bloodstream is taken up by muscles, so let's focus on those cells.

Fat droplets called diacylglycerol have been studied extensively by researchers at Yale University using advanced techniques to image muscles with MRI technology.[5] In a person still producing insulin in the pancreas (all but type 1 diabetics), as blood sugar rises after a meal, insulin is released into the bloodstream from the pancreas. Insulin circulates and arrives at muscle cells where the glucose can be used for energy or stored. However, if the muscle cell is toxic with fat droplets, a condition called lipotoxicity, then the insulin does not as readily initiate a series of steps via its receptor that ideally result in glucose leaving the bloodstream and entering the muscle cell. This delay in removing glucose from the blood is known as insulin resistance, or IR, which we talked about before. The blood glucose remains high, and the potential for untoward reactions of an elevated glucose on arteries, nerves, kidney cells, the brain, and so on can begin. The key to reversing IR found in type 2 diabetes is to reverse the lipotoxicity brought about by the fat droplets. The low-fat diets used by Marc and Robby and in many research studies have been shown to reverse the IR and therefore the severity or very presence of type 2 diabetes. Get the fat out, and the insulin will work again. It will work for you.

What both Marc and Robby (see the case studies above) have been able to do by lowering their overall dietary fat content, and particularly their dietary saturated fat content, is to reduce and reverse the amount of lipotoxic fats clogging their muscle cells. This permits the most efficient insulin signaling possible, whether the insulin is made naturally in Marc or is injected by Robby. Your cells work the same way and will respond in the same manner. Do what they did and get what they got.

Feed the Microbiome

We have much to learn about which specific foods boost the microbiome to protect against insulin resistance the most. For now, eat plants, not animals, and avoid added oil. Foods that feed healthy bacterial colonies include asparagus, garlic, Jerusalem artichokes, jicama, and onions.

Study In-Depth: The Plant-Based Solution Versus the American Diabetes Association Diet

Do you know the GEICO lizard in TV ads? It may well be that the reason he is so thin is that Dr. Neal Barnard is in charge of making sure employees of that company have plant-based options at work that prevent and reverse type 2 diabetes.

Dr. Barnard has been a leader in performing scientific studies to assess the effectiveness of plant-based diets. Although he grew up in farming country of North Dakota, his job during school helping perform autopsies made a big impact. He saw the clogged arteries that looked like animal fat, and he put one and one together to change his diet away from animal products.

Barnard trained as a psychiatrist, but his career transformed when he founded the Physicians Committee for Responsible Medicine. One project was the publication of a twenty-two-week study of the impact of a low-fat, plant-based vegan diet. In this study, ninety-nine individuals with type 2 diabetes followed either a plant-based diet or a diet based on the American Diabetes Association (ADA) guidelines for twenty-two weeks. The vegan diet (made up of approximately 10 percent fat, 15 percent protein, and 75 percent carbohydrate) consisted of vegetables, fruits, grains, and legumes. Participants were asked to avoid animal products and added fats and to favor foods that cause a lower and slower rise in blood-sugar levels (also known as low-glycemic-index foods), such as beans and green vegetables. Portion sizes, energy intake, and carbohydrate intake were unrestricted.[6]

By the end of the study, 43 percent of the plant-based and even 26 percent of the ADA group were able to reduce doses of diabetic medications. All the participants got a lot of attention, which may have helped both groups. The HgbA1C (see "Monitoring Diabetes" sidebar above) fell by 1.23 percent in the vegan group versus 0.38 in the ADA group, indicating more normal blood sugars in the vegan group. Body weight fell by over thirteen pounds in the vegan group versus six to seven pounds in the other group. Finally, blood LDL ("bad") cholesterol and the leakage of protein into the urine fell more in the vegan study group. This indicates better artery health. Dr. Barnard has studied a plant-based diet in the cafeterias at GEICO offices and found the same benefits.

It is likely that the low-fat, plant-based diet influenced nutrition and body composition in several ways. First, plant-based diets are more nutrient dense, and weight loss is accelerated. Second, reductions in dietary fat, particularly saturated fat, may increase insulin sensitivity by presumably reducing the muscle cell lipotoxicity (toxicity due to too much fat). Finally, plant-based diets provide dietary iron in a different form called non-heme iron, and that may also facilitate insulin sensitivity. Whatever is the exact pathway or pathways, eat plants not animals and do not add oils. Isn't it amazing that you do not just have to manage your type 2 diabetes but you can eliminate it?

Associations Between Eating Meat and Diabetes

There is research that suggests that meat can cause insulin resistance (whereby cells can't properly absorb glucose from the bloodstream) and type 2 diabetes. I want you to know about several findings, which link eating meat and developing diabetes mellitus, that should make you love your plants.

1. In 1985, the risk of diabetes was analyzed in 25,000 vegetarians and meat eaters. The study found that women who ate red meat increased their risk of developing diabetes by 40 percent and men who ate red meat increased their risk by 80 percent.[7]

2. In 2008, a study looked at over 8,000 Seventh-day Adventists and found that meat eaters had a 74 percent increase in the development of diabetes.[8]

3. In 2009, 61,000 people were examined, and results showed that meat eaters were twice as likely to develop diabetes as those who were totally plant-based.[9]

4. In a study of meat and diabetes, scientists found that for every 3.5 ounces of red meat consumed per day, diabetes risk increased 10 percent. And for every 1.75 ounces of processed red meat consumed per day (about the equivalent of one packaged hot dog), the risk increased 51 percent.[10] On a positive note, researchers also found that the risk for developing type 2 diabetes dropped significantly when people swapped a serving of meat for a serving of nuts.

5. The results of a large study published in the journal *Diabetologia* showed that eating processed red meat (bacon, salami, hot dogs, lunch meats) more than five times a week increased the risk of diabetes by 91 percent, and eating red meat increased it by 59 percent.[11]

6. The same study written up in *Diabetologia* found that every 10 grams of animal protein consumed daily increased the risk of diabetes by 6 percent. (Keep in mind that 100 grams is 3.5 ounces, so this is a small amount.)[12]

7. In a massive analysis involving 195,000 participants, diabetes risk went up with the number of times fish was consumed weekly.[13]

Although theses associations do not prove that meat causes diabetes, as other factors may be shared by meat eaters, there is ample reason to suspect that the link between animal products and diabetes is real. In group comparisons, meat eaters are heavier than those who don't eat meat; they also consume less fiber and consume more dietary fat. Increases in body weight, particularly around the abdomen (called visceral fat), are pro-inflammatory. Inflammation is linked to type 2 diabetes. Finally, meat-based diets can also have excess amounts of the pro-oxidant iron and preservatives, like nitrates, which damage tissues and result in insulin resistance. So what else does meat have that may mess with diabetes?

Seven More Drawbacks of Meat

I really want you to ditch all meat products as soon as possible, so I am going to open your eyes to more of the risks associated with consuming meat. Meat creates a series of reactions that favor not only diabetes but also heart disease and cancer. Here are seven scientifically proven harmful chemicals associated with eating meat that are rarely discussed. You do not want these chemicals marinating your brain and body.

1. HIGH-SENSITIVITY C-REACTIVE PROTEIN (HS-CRP)

Inflammation can be helpful when we have a mosquito bite, and the redness, swelling, and pain indicate that our immune system is fighting back to clean up the area. Inflammation is not desirable, however, as a chronic condition due to our lifestyle or environment and can lead to chronic diseases. One way to assess for chronic inflammation is to measure a chemical in the blood made by the liver called hs-CRP. This chemical is produced during inflammation and predicts the development of serious illness, including cardiovascular disease and diabetes mellitus. Multiple studies have found that, even after correcting for confounding factors, meat consumption is associated with elevated hs-CRP.[14] In other words, it's a scientific fact that meat is inflammatory. This has not received enough attention!

2. INSULIN

Insulin release varies according to what foods we are eating. Scientists have looked at how eating certain foods affects the release of insulin.[15] Surprisingly, some protein-rich and fat-rich foods (eggs, beef, fish, cheese) induced as much insulin secretion as did some carbohydrate-rich foods (beef was equal to brown rice, and fish was equal to bread).

The researchers found that fish, beef, cheese, and eggs resulted in larger insulin responses per gram than many carbohydrate foods. The scientific fact that meat stimulates insulin production is rarely mentioned. Higher insulin levels from animal products can compound the high insulin levels from eating a high-fat diet of any kind and the subsequent insulin resistance.

3. INSULIN-LIKE GROWTH FACTOR 1 (IGF-1)

IGF-1 is a peptide hormone that stimulates cell growth. It's also linked to breast and prostate cancers. Meat eaters consistently have higher levels of IGF-1.[16] What's more interesting is that breast and prostate cancers are rare in traditional Asian communities, which have a very low intake of animal products. For example, among Okinawans (traditionally some of the longest-living people on the planet), meat makes up less than 10 percent of their daily calories, and both diabetes and cancer are very rare.

4. METHIONINE

Methionine is an amino acid found largely in animal products. Consuming less methionine is associated with increased lifespan. Getting too much methionine can create oxidative stress and mitochondrial damage, which are common pathologies in diabetes mellitus. Vegan diets tend to be relatively low in methionine and to have low rates of diabetes.[17]

5. TRIMETHYLAMINE N-OXIDE (TMAO)

Recall from the prior chapter that TMAO is produced by intestinal bacteria as a result of our dietary choices. Levels of TMAO, which have been shown to increase plaque buildup in the arteries, are now routinely measured in patients in my clinic and go down when eggs and meat are avoided. Higher levels of TMAO in patients with diabetes mellitus predict a worrisome prognosis for the future with double the number of cardiac events and death.[18] Eating a plant-based diet generally insures low levels of TMAO.

6. PERSISTENT ORGANIC POLLUTANTS (POPS)

POPs are toxic synthetic chemicals that accumulate in fat. The best known ones are PCBs, dioxins, DDT, and flame retardants used in clothing and furniture. They disrupt endocrine pathways and are linked to many chronic diseases.[19] Where do POPs come from? Largely from the meat that we eat. For example, levels of PCBs in animal fat, cow's milk, butter, and fish are much, much higher than the levels found in vegetables, fruits, and cereals. Although all of us are exposed to environmental toxins and chemical pollutants, the Plant-Based Solution protects us from the high levels usually sourced from animal-rich diets.

7. ADVANCED GLYCATION END PRODUCTS (AGES)

AGEs are naturally present compounds in food and can be increased by cooking on dry heat, such as on a grill. AGEs are associated with a variety of diseases, including brain inflammation, diabetes, heart disease, and cancer.[20] Levels of AGEs found in meat and cheese are many multiples higher than in any fruit or vegetable. Increased levels of AGEs lead to premature aging and diabetes and are best avoided. There is no easy way to measure the amount of AGEs in your body, but the diabetic test HgbA1C may reflect the process. Nondiabetics and former diabetics will generally have lower amounts. When you adopt the Plant-Based Solution, you are also adopting an eating pattern that is very low in AGEs compared to a diet that includes meat, eggs, and dairy.

Know Your Insulin Level

Insulin is produced in the pancreas and helps the body turn sugar into energy. Too much insulin can result in lower HDL ("good") cholesterol levels and higher LDL ("bad") cholesterol levels. Excess insulin can also lead to insulin resistance, reduced magnesium levels, and inflammation. Weight gain is also a side effect of excess insulin because too much insulin encourages the body to store fat.

Insulin is commonly measured in microunits per milliliter (mcU/ml). According to University of Washington researcher Stephan Guyenet, PhD, "The average insulin level in the United States is 8.8 mIU/ml for men and 8.4 for women. Given the degree of metabolic dysfunction in this country, I think it's safe to say that the ideal level of fasting insulin is probably below 8.4 uIU/mL . . . [Best] would be 2–6."[21]

Have your fasting insulin level measured the next time you see your doctor.

Plant-Based Diets Can Reverse Diabetic Neuropathy

While there are many concerns associated with the diagnosis of diabetes, one of the most distressing to patients is the development of diabetic neuropathy. This may be a minor tingling in the hands and feet (stocking-glove distribution, as it is called) but can progress to pain, loss of feeling, and injury to joints. Neuropathy can also involve nerves feeding the heart, stomach, and blood vessels, and then it is called autonomic neuropathy. This is a very serious condition when it develops. I published several studies on this condition when I was a resident physician.

I have already praised Dr. Neal Barnard for his important research, but he also deserves appreciation for a recently completed study that he conducted with other researchers on adopting a low-fat vegan diet for diabetic neuropathy.[22] Patients with type 2 diabetes and painful neuropathy were assigned to two diet groups. One followed their usual diet while the other adopted a low-fat, plant-based diet for twenty weeks. Both groups took vitamin B12 supplements. The plant-based group lost weight, about thirteen pounds, even though calories were not restricted. Measurements of nerve function in the skin improved during the plant-based diet. Measures of pain also improved during the study period. Although the researchers considered their findings a pilot study, it is hopeful that even advanced complications of type 2 diabetes, like nerve damage, respond in a relatively short time span to the Plant-Based Solution. If you are dealing with neuropathy—or do not want to deal with it—stick to a plant diet starting today.

CASE STUDY

Goodbye Diabetes Is Music to the Ear

Bill is a well-known musician who developed heart disease and needed a coronary bypass operation before I met him. He had struggled with type 2 diabetes related to his obesity for years. He played events late at night, and his diet was a typical Western one, with many fast-food meals. I met him seven years after his heart surgery and introduced him to the concept of diabetes reversal with plant-based diets. He had never heard of such a possibility and got very excited. He read books, watched videos, and began attending the Plant Based Nutrition Support Group meetings. The initial challenge, which he shared with me in my office, was finding enough diet-compliant foods that he'd enjoy. Here's what Bill said:

> I converted to plant-based eating in stages, over a few months, the first stage being eating meat just once a week. Daily tracking of my ongoing weight loss and drop in blood-sugar numbers provided continuing motivation. In a little over two months, my blood sugar remained in the 80s to 90s range (much better results and more normal than before the diet change), and I was able to discontinue my insulin. Blood work at my doctor's office also indicated my total cholesterol had dropped over 100 points, and my triglycerides level was cut in half! I also lost over thirty-five pounds, which gave me renewed energy and a new outlook on life! Plant-based eating has provided a cure—not just a management program— for diabetes!

Bill has remained off all medications for diabetes for over three years and has a renewed energy and spirit that confirms the power of the Plant-Based Solution. By reading and sharing this book, and by putting the knowledge and power of your plate into action now, you do not need to be trapped in the world of pills and procedures. ■

Seventh-day Adventists Are Plant-Based Heroes

Loma Linda, California, is a very special and important city for you to know about. One of the most compelling reasons to choose a plant-based eating pattern to prevent, manage, or reverse diabetes comes from a massive database derived from the Seventh-day Adventist Church (SDA), headquartered in Loma Linda. A religious principle of the SDA church is to eat a vegetarian diet. About half of SDA followers do that to some degree, with about 10 percent choosing a vegan diet.

The official doctrine of the church is that members are called upon to care for their bodies, treating them with the respect a divine creation deserves. Gluttony and excess, even of something good, is considered detrimental to health. Their beliefs are that a well-balanced vegetarian diet that avoids the consumption of meat coupled with the intake of legumes, whole grains, nuts, fruits, and vegetables, along with a source of vitamin B12, promotes vigorous health.

Beginning in 1958, scientists have taken detailed diet histories and followed the health of tens of thousands of SDA members. Because the SDA members are similar in many other respects, they have provided a valuable natural experiment in diet and health. The groundbreaking research, called the Adventist Health Study, has yielded a series of research projects and publications on the links between diet, lifestyle, disease, and mortality of church members. There are few studies that are this large, this carefully tracked, and with long-term follow-up. Several important observations have been published in peer-reviewed publications from a phase of the study involving over 96,000 men and women in the SDA church. The findings relate to the risk of diabetes and other diseases.

Five powerful takeaways from the results of the Adventist Health Study are:

1. **Vegetarians are diagnosed with diabetes far less often than non-vegetarians.** Over 41,000 SDA participants were followed for diabetes. During follow-up, over 2 percent of non-vegetarians developed diabetes compared with 0.5 percent of vegans and approximately 1 percent of other vegetarian types.

2. **Vegetarians live longer than non-vegetarians.** An earlier phase of the SDA study found that eating a vegetarian diet with plenty of nuts added five years to one's life. Simply put, vegetarians lived longer than non-vegetarians in the SDA population. SDA members who consumed fish had the lowest mortality, followed by vegans and lacto-ovo vegetarians (milk and egg eaters) and finally, the meat eaters.

3. **Vegetarians have lower cancer rates than non-vegetarians.** In the same SDA study, cancer rates were available for over 69,000 of the study members. Cancer risk was significantly lower among vegetarians, with vegans having by far the lowest risk of cancer.

4. **Vegetarians are less likely to die of heart disease than non-vegetarians.** In the full group of over 96,000 participants, vegetarians enjoyed great freedom from deaths due to cardiovascular disease, with a 50 percent reduction in vegan men. Longer follow-up of women will be needed, as they enjoy lower overall heart death rates at the average age of the SDA study.

5. **Vegetarians have lower blood pressure than non-vegetarians.** In a sub-study of white and black SDA populations, average blood pressure was lower for vegetarians and was the lowest of all for vegans.

It is important to realize that the Adventist Health Study is not a randomized diet study (a randomized study is one in which participants are randomly allocated to either the group receiving treatment or the control group). I doubt there will ever be a study this large and for this long performed in a randomized manner. Therefore, for those determined to live healthy lives, the Adventist Health Study provides lessons to guide choices for optimal health.

I want to leave you with the words of Dr. Dean Ornish, who demonstrated the reversal of heart disease. He said, "Think about it: Heart disease and diabetes, which account for more deaths in the U.S. and worldwide than everything else combined, are completely preventable by making comprehensive lifestyle changes. Without drugs or surgery."[23]

Plant Rant

The trend to prescribe LCHF (low-carbohydrate, high-fat) diets for diabetic patients, sometimes patterned as a Paleo diet, has grown in the headlines and occasionally small clinical studies with short follow-up. Diets that omit processed foods and dairy are better diets than the standard Western junk fare. The studies on LCHF diets often make headlines perhaps due to the powerful presence of the meat and dairy industries that can advertise heavily and stand to benefit from the confusion.

Those who promote the widespread adoption of LCHF diets for diabetes rarely, if ever, mention that the long-term results of LCHF diets in large studies include increased mortality, a rather heavy penalty.[24] Plant-based diets are the answer to diabetic health while also advancing the health of the earth and the lives of billions of animals otherwise forced to suffer horrible lives.

THE PLANT-BASED PLAN   **Today, Stop the Soda Habit**

Choose a naturally sugar-free beverage instead: flavored sparkling water; homemade iced tea (green tea and herbal teas work well), unsweetened or with stevia; water with a squeeze of citrus; or kombucha (fermented tea).

4

Slim and Trim

Measuring the weight of the nation or considering your weight is not necessarily a comment on whether skinny or portly looks better. Rather, it is a fact that your body weight serves as a relatively easy measure of a potential host of problems. Without question, diabetes, high blood pressure, certain cancers, dementia, arthritis, and heart disease afflict more people who are obese. To decrease your risk of chronic illness, to lower your health-care costs, and to enjoy the best odds of avoiding illness and hospitalizations, we have to talk about your weight.

The Centers for Disease Control has been publishing state-by-state graphs of the number of obese citizens as a percentage of the total population since 1985. When I began practice in 1990, only one state classified over 20 percent of its adult population as obese (Mississippi). Now there are only five states with 20–25 percent obesity, with all others being higher than that![1] In fact, four states, all southern, now have more than 35 percent of the adult population obese. Louisiana holds the ominous title of the most obese state with 36 percent. Obesity exceeds 30 percent of the adult population in half of the states in the United States.

The equation for why obesity is skyrocketing is complex. The widespread availability of cheap processed foods in stores, fast-food restaurants, school vending machines, and even hospitals and gyms is surely a major part of the problem. Sedentary lifestyles, where people are glued to smartphones, tablets, and game stations, is another big piece of the problem. Environmental toxins from plastics, pollution, linings of cans and fast-food containers, and other sources is part of it by introducing endocrine-disrupting chemicals into the bodies of young children. Poor sleep contributes to some of the problem. Stress is a factor too.

While the cause of the rise of obesity is complex, a solution that is supported by a large and robust amount of literature is the Plant-Based Solution. This is truly a secret that needs to be shared. The solution is in the produce department at your local grocer. The Plant-Based Solution can return your waistline to a healthier and smaller state. But will it work for you? It worked very well for Allan.

CASE STUDY

The Round Podiatrist Who Learned to Run

I have known Allan for over forty years. We grew up in the same neighborhood a few years apart. I went on to medical school, and Allan pursued training in podiatry. Over the years, we lost touch but reconnected on social media. Since we had been in contact many years earlier, Allan's weight had increased to 284 pounds on a five-foot, seven-inch frame. His joints ached from the statin drugs he was using to lower his cholesterol, he was winded walking up a flight of stairs, and he was taking blood pressure medicine daily. He wore a mask on his face at night for sleep apnea. He knew he was on a path to disaster and was looking for a way out that would work long term. Allan decided to make a New Year's resolution and go for a health change after reading my social media posts every day praising the Plant-Based Solution. He bought a vegan cookbook and a few new items like kale, quinoa, steel-cut oats, and farro, and Allan started cooking.

When I last talked with Allan, he said, "It's coming up on three years now, and I have lost 110 pounds. My waist is thirty-two inches, and my shirts are now M instead of XXL. I am off statins, and my cholesterol is 137. No more blood pressure pills. No more need to wear a CPAP mask for sleep apnea either. I had an overnight sleep study done, and my sleep apnea has disappeared. After losing about 100 pounds, I started running. I got my distance up to 5K and have moved that to 10K distances. I kind of look forward to it now." Allan's low cholesterol level is impressive and meaningful because several doctors, including world-famous pathologist William Roberts and Cleveland Clinic legend Caldwell Esselstyn, indicate that a total cholesterol under 150 mg/dl, like Allan's, can make you essentially heart attack proof. Good job, Allan.

Allan has also begun writing a blog that includes simple recipes he prepares that are plant-based and oil-free. His renewed energy and his commitment to health and weight loss using natural methods have made him a local hero who inspires many to follow his path. I am certain he will never return to an obese body size because he had the willpower to change and found that simple, plant-based cooking allowed him the skill to succeed. Allan is a vegan badass, and I am in awe of the changes he has made. But he will tell you, if he could do it, you can do it too. ■

Study In-Depth: The National Cholesterol Education Program Diet Versus a Vegan Diet

Can you really trust the science that the Plant-Based Solution is the answer to your weight issues? You may recall the name Neal Barnard, of the Physicians Committee for Responsible Medicine, for his original research, which was highlighted in the previous chapter. Dr. Barnard contributed to another landmark paper regarding plant-based nutrition, this time on long-term weight loss.[2] Sixty-two overweight, post-menopausal women followed a plant-based diet for fourteen weeks. Individuals in the vegan group lost more weight than those who followed a diet endorsed by the National Cholesterol Education Program (NCEP) at one year (eleven pounds versus four pounds) and at two years (seven pounds versus two pounds). The participants who were offered group support lost more weight at one year and two years than those without support. Attendance at meetings was associated with improved weight loss at one year and two years.

The authors concluded that a vegan diet was associated with significantly greater weight loss than the NCEP diet at one and two years. Both group support and meeting attendance were associated with significant weight loss at follow-up. This is science at its best. A tough problem, a well-designed study, and meaningful results. If you will ditch the meat, add the veggies, and get some friends doing the same, you will see your waistline decrease. And wouldn't that feel nice?

Science Corner: Plants and Weight

If you need more data that eliminating animal products and eating exclusively plant foods can control your waistline, let me tell you about another study conducted by Neal Barnard and other researchers. Dr. Barnard and his team performed a randomized study of diet and weight loss, this time in a work setting.[3] Employees from ten sites of the GEICO insurance company who were either overweight or had a diagnosis of diabetes followed a low-fat vegan diet with weekly group support and work cafeteria options available for eighteen weeks. Mean body weight fell six pounds in the low-fat vegan group and not at all in the control group. Along with the weight loss, the low-fat vegan diet resulted in lower cholesterol and blood sugar. The people who completed the study to the very end lost even more weight overall.

You can actually use your work site as a place to kick off your plant-based health plan. All you have to do is develop the habit of packing low-fat, plant-based meals in your lunchbox and you may be on your way to a slimmer waistline. Get a group to do it with you and your success increases.

More Proof That a Plant-Based Diet Leads to Weight Loss

A meta-analysis is a research technique that combines several similar studies and analyzes the overall results, which are larger and may be more powerful. A meta-analysis was performed on twelve randomized studies of weight loss involving 1,151 subjects who were studied on average for eighteen weeks.[4] Subjects assigned to vegetarian diets lost more weight than those assigned to non-vegetarian diets, with the most weight loss in those eating a vegan diet (five to six pounds). Of course, studies that limited calories showed more weight loss overall.

In another study designed to examine the role of plant-based diets on weight loss, five different diets were compared for six months.[5] Overweight adults between the ages of eighteen and sixty-five were put on a low-fat, low–glycemic index diet that was either vegan, vegetarian, pesco-vegetarian (fish and plants), semi-vegetarian, or omnivorous. At six months, the weight loss in the vegan group (sixteen pounds) was significantly greater than the other groups. Vegan participants also decreased their fat and saturated fat more than the pesco-vegetarian, semi-vegetarian, and omnivorous groups. The study indicated that vegan diets may result in greater weight loss than more modest recommendations.

Let's turn again now to that very special church in Loma Linda, the SDA, and healthy diets. Researchers assessed the body-mass index (BMI), which is used as a measure of body weight, of 22,434 members of the SDA Adventist Health Study. Normal BMI is between about 18 and 25. BMI was lowest in vegans (a score of 24), higher in lacto-ovo vegetarians (26), higher yet in pesco-vegetarians (26.3), climbing more in semi-vegetarians (27), and peaked out (29) in non-vegetarians.[6] These data strongly suggest that a nutrient-dense, plant-based diet is the best path to sustained weight loss and management.

CASE STUDY

The Comedian Who Laughed Last

Comedian and magician Penn Jillette, of Penn and Teller, knew he was in trouble. Despite his six-foot, seven-inch frame, the Vegas headliner weighed 330 pounds, and his blood pressure was spiking, which sent him repeatedly to the emergency room. He was facing bariatric surgery as he approached his sixtieth birthday. He realized that extreme results would require extreme measures, so he adopted a plant-based diet of about 1,000 calories a day and lost just under one pound a day. He ate no animal products, no processed grains, and no added sugar or salt. He patterned his weight loss after the program of Dr. Joel Fuhrman, stressing nutrient-dense foods, but took it further than most. He ate only potatoes for two weeks but then added in large amounts of spinach, oranges, blueberries, cayenne pepper, and cacao powder.

Jillette got what he wanted from his weight loss: he's healthier and lost over 100 pounds without surgery. He has kept it off for over a year and allows himself to splurge a bit once every two weeks. He has managed to make the plant-based diet work on the road and has restaurants prepare him simple plant-based meals without oil. Although most of us do not need to lose over 100 pounds, the results obtained by Jillette are a reminder that if you take away the foods that inflame and irritate the body and replace them with WFPB foods, the body will tend to heal itself.[7] ■

Plant Rant

Diets patterned after the Atkins plan, using low-carbohydrate, high-fat eating patterns, can lead to short-term weight loss in studies. Trading short-term weight loss for the long-term adverse consequences of LCHF diets, including reports of increased death rates, is simply not reasonable or advisable. The Adventist Health Study makes the point that vegan diets win the race for the best dietary pattern for long-term weight management. It is the dietary pattern you should adopt.

THE PLANT-BASED PLAN **Build Your Snack Arsenal**

Having a variety of healthy snacks available can set you up for success on your plant-based diet, especially when you are transitioning. Plan ahead to have healthy options available, so you aren't tempted by something simply because it's easy:

- Apple or banana with nut or seed butter

- Hummus with gluten-free crackers or veggies

- Celery with nut butter and raisins

- Smoothie

- Frozen grapes

- Granola and plant milk

- A handful of nuts and a piece of fruit

- Crispy chickpeas: drained and rinsed chickpeas, tossed with olive oil and salt, baked until crunchy (about 1 hour)

- Kale chips: destemmed, torn curly kale leaves, tossed with olive oil and salt, baked until crisp (about 20 minutes)

- Energy balls: In a food processor mix 1 cup pitted dates; $2/3$ cup oats; 3 tablespoons nut or seed butter; 1 tablespoon chia, hemp, or ground flax seeds. Stir in ¼ cup chocolate chips or cacao nibs. Roll into golf-ball-sized rounds. Refrigerate.

- Tortilla chips and guacamole or salsa

- Store-bought options: seaweed snacks; individually packaged nut butters; baked plantain chips; granola bars; banana, apple, or kale chips

5

High on Plants for
Low Blood Pressure

E levated blood pressure, or hypertension, as it's more commonly known in the halls of hospitals, is a real big deal, and you may be dealing with it. My office is full of patients with high blood pressure. This killer is often silent, like the early stages of clogged heart arteries and prediabetes, so you might have it right now and not know it.

Hypertension is a serious problem. In the United States alone, about 1,000 deaths every day involve high blood pressure as a primary or contributing cause.[1] Most people suffering a heart attack have hypertension. Almost all stroke victims have high blood pressure. Most patients with kidney failure have hypertension. And most people with congestive heart failure have high blood pressure.

On a global basis, hypertension is a huge issue too. A study called the Global Burden of Disease (GBD) was initiated in 1992 as a collaborative effort between the World Bank and the World Health Organization. The GBD 2010 study had a number of important findings with respect to high blood pressure around the world. High blood pressure ranked as the single leading risk factor for disease. High blood pressure went from being the fourth-leading risk factor in 1990 for GBD to the number-one risk factor in 2010.[2]

Nobel Prize-Winning Science:
Plants in Your Mouth Lower Blood Pressure

When you sit down to eat a meal, you might not be thinking about the Nobel Prize, but you can thank the recipients of this award to help you improve your blood pressure. The 1998 Nobel Prize in Medicine was awarded to three researchers for describing the central role of nitric oxide, or NO, as a signaling molecule in the cardiovascular system (discussed in chapter 2). When arteries make a lot of NO, blood pressure tends to be in the normal range. NO production improves when you adopt healthy lifestyle measures such as eating a lot of fruit and vegetables, along with avoiding smoking and getting regular exercise. Foods rich in polyphenols, including apples and grapes, can activate the enzyme that produces NO. An apple a day and a bunch of grapes may keep your blood pressure medicine away.

Another pathway based on plant-based diets that boosts NO production in your arteries has drawn much attention in the past few years. Leafy greens and some other vegetables, like beets, are rich in dietary nitrates. These are not the nitrates found in bacon and pepperoni, so you still have to ditch those to be healthy. When you chew greens and beets, the dietary nitrates interact with hidden bacteria in the grooves of your tongue and get converted to nitrites. When the nitrates are swallowed, they are absorbed into the blood and are converted to NO by enzymes waiting for you to feed them healthy substrates. Even if you swallow these nitrate-rich vegetables, like kale and beets, in juice or a smoothie—with little time to settle on your tongue—the dietary nitrates are rapidly absorbed in your GI tract and appear in your bloodstream.

This next step is so cool. These nitrates, which have not been chewed much and have not mixed with the bacteria on your tongue, concentrate in your salivary glands, the parotid glands. There they are excreted into your saliva, which then coats your tongue and has time to interact with those hungry bacteria. On this second pass through your body, the dietary nitrates get converted to NO. The green drink you swallowed forty-five minutes ago may be secreted right onto your tongue to enjoy the bacteria-nitrate interaction. In other words, if the bacteria doesn't get to your dietary nitrates the first time down, this "entero-salivary" recirculation makes sure they get them the second time around. Is that not amazing? The recirculation of nitrates to produce NO is a reason to embrace the Plant-Based Solution by packing in WFPB choices that you chew or drink several times a day. The new advice from a doctor to a patient might as well be, "A kale salad a day keeps the doctor away."

Study In-Depth: Eat Your Plants to Lower Blood Pressure

You read about the Adventist Health Study, which offers a large and long-term look at dietary patterns and the associations with health and disease. Associations do not always prove that the topic studied, in this case dietary style, resulted in the outcome. However, when studying the Adventists and seeing that the rates of type 2 diabetes, obesity, and cancers are the lowest of any eating style, it is highly likely that it is cause and effect.

In a study that analyzed 592 subjects, 25 percent were either vegan or lacto-ovo vegetarians (labeled "vegetarian/vegans"), 13 percent were pesco-vegetarian, and 62 percent were non-vegetarian.[3] Compared with non-vegetarians, the vegetarian/vegans had "odds ratios" for hypertension of 0.56, meaning hypertension was present in about half of them. That constitutes a huge reduction in the risk for hypertension-related cardiovascular disease.

Why are plant-based diets associated with less hypertension? You know about plant-based foods and NO production. Another possibility is that plant-based diets provide greater intakes of potassium, other minerals (like magnesium), and fiber, which may all lower blood pressure. It is also possible that meat increases the risk of hypertension because of its association with fewer vegetables and fruits in the diet and the potential for more inflammation. The lower BMI among many vegetarians may help. Plant foods are also known to protect against insulin resistance, which in turn is related to hypertension and other risk factors for heart disease. There are so many potential ways the Plant-Based Solution may lower your blood pressure.

CASE STUDY
Goodbye Blood Pressure Medicine with Plants

Cheryl is a beautiful woman. At age fifty-five, she will catch your eye. But she has had a few bumps in the health road. She developed chest pains and was found to have serious heart artery blockages in her late forties, requiring heart bypass surgery. She had been on blood pressure medications for twenty years, and her father had heart disease. She did not smoke but worked in smoking environments.

When she began seeing me, I was struck by her warm heart and kind nature. I introduced her to the science of plant-based heart therapy, and she announced a goal of getting off many medications—at the time, she was taking thirteen prescription drugs. For a year she tried to follow a fully plant-based diet but went on and off it around holidays and when facing other common obstacles.

Over a year ago she decided to fully commit to eating a low-fat WFPB diet as part of the Plant-Based Solution. The results followed. Her weight began to decrease, and she has lost over twenty pounds but is never hungry, as nutrient-dense foods fill her up faster than fast foods. Her cholesterol has responded as well as her blood pressure. She has been able to reduce the number of prescription medications from thirteen to three. She has energy, sleeps well, enjoys her job (now out of a smoking area), and teaches others the power of the plate for blood pressure control. She has a new attitude, empowered by controlling her own health destiny, and a boyfriend too! It is startling how making the decision to treat your body as the miracle that it is can improve so many measures of health. Cheryl is an amazing miracle herself. She knows that if she could do it, so can you. ■

Hot Question: Do Vegans Need Supplements?

Despite all the benefits of a plant-based diet described in this book, there are supplements that vegans should take and some they might consider taking. Remember, those eating animal-rich diets often take "supplements" called *insulin, statins,* and *chemotherapy.* A few vitamins are no big deal compared with those.

VITAMIN B12

Vitamin B12 is important in brain, nerve, and hematologic health and is a factor in a key process called "methylation," which regulates levels of homocysteine (high levels are associated with heart disease risk). It's well known that animal products are richer in vitamin B12 than plants. Actually, neither plants nor animals make B12. It's produced by bacteria that reside in the gastrointestinal tract of animals other than humans. When animal products are eaten, B12 is ingested as a bystander.

By some estimates, 50 percent of vegans and 10 percent of vegetarians are deficient in vitamin B12. I recommend taking about 2,500 mcg once a week of vitamin B12, ideally as a liquid, sublingual, or chewable form for better absorption, or 500 mcg daily if that schedule works better for you.

VITAMIN D

Vitamin D is known to promote bone health but is also proving to be essential in blood pressure and blood glucose control, in heart function, and in brain function. Measurements of blood levels are the best way to assess adequacy of vitamin D. Vegans tend to have lower levels of vitamin D.

Direct sunshine on exposed skin for twenty to thirty minutes a day can provide adequate vitamin D, but for many people oral supplementation is necessary to reach proper blood levels. Vitamin D3 is the form most commonly recommended but is usually derived from animal sources such as lanolin. If this is not acceptable, vegan versions of vitamin D3 are available. Vitamin D2 comes from plant sources, mushrooms being a rich source, but is not as reliably absorbed. While the standard recommendation is to supplement with 800 IU a day, I suggest 2,000 IU of D3 a day.

OMEGA-3

Omega-3 is an important essential fatty acid that in adequate supply helps control inflammation, supports healthy brain function and growth, and contributes to normal blood sugar, blood pressure, and cholesterol levels. Most recognize salmon, sardines, and herring as cold-water fish that can supply these fatty acids directly. However, these fish come with the burden of cholesterol, saturated fats, and potential contamination from mercury and persistent organic pollutants like PCBs. Many of my patients who eat fish have elevated blood-mercury levels, some very high. Ground flax seed as a source of alpha-linolenic acid, or ALA, is recommended in a dose of about two tablespoons daily along with three halves of English walnuts. Beyond this, it may be wise to take algae-based vegan DHA and EPA. I recommend about 250 mg of plant-based EPA/DHA in a capsule form, which is widely available.

IODINE

For those who don't enjoy sea vegetables, like seaweed or dulce, a 150 mcg a day supplement of iodine is an option.

Science Corner: Vegans Have the Lowest Blood Pressures

If you are looking for more support that your plant-based choices in the grocery store and farmers market can prevent or reverse blood pressure problems, there is more. The Adventist Health Study did additional studies relating dietary choices to blood pressure diagnoses and this time analyzed a subset of white subjects.[4] In 500 subjects studied, the vegan/vegetarians had blood pressure lower than omnivorous Adventists. The vegans were also less likely to be using blood pressure medications. The odds ratio for being diagnosed with high blood pressure or taking a blood pressure medication was reduced by 70 percent in the plant-based eaters! This is a huge number that would translate to hundreds of thousands of lives saved yearly in the United States alone.

Two more studies are worthy of consideration. The first is a study of the power of adopting a low-fat vegan diet for only seven days. Most anyone could eat a plant-based diet without oil for seven days, right? Dr. John McDougall, MD, deserves his reputation as a giant and legend in the plant-based medical world. He has been teaching a starch-based low-fat diet for over forty years and runs a popular and effective treatment center in Santa Rosa, California.

Dr. McDougall recently published the results of over 1,600 participants who came to his program for a one-week immersion.[5] In a hotel setting, attendees were provided meals that were low-fat (≤10 percent of calories), high carbohydrate (~80 percent of calories), moderate sodium, and purely plant-based for seven days. They all had measures of health assessed, including blood pressure, before and after the week by trained medical professionals. The results showed that even though most blood pressure medications were reduced or discontinued at baseline, systolic blood pressure (the top blood pressure number) decreased by a median 8 mmHg and diastolic blood pressure (the bottom number) by 4 mmHg during the week. These are quite remarkable findings in such a large database. Participants lost an average of three pounds and also had improvements in blood sugar and cholesterol. Patients finished the program at substantially lower predicted heart risk than when they arrived a week earlier, a powerful result.

The second study of note comes from Europe and is called the EPIC-Oxford study. In this major study of nutrition and health, researchers analyzed the impact of dietary patterns and hypertension.[6] In the United Kingdom, 11,004 men and women aged twenty to seventy-eight reported on whether they had blood pressure problems and filled out dietary surveys. Self-reported hypertension ranged from 15 percent in male meat eaters to 5.8 percent in male vegans, nearly three times as high in the meat eaters! Hypertension was reported in 12.1 percent of female meat eaters and 7.7 percent in female vegans. Fish eaters and vegetarians had similar rates of hypertension, which were about halfway between the meat eaters and vegans.

Participants had their blood pressure measured. Systolic and diastolic blood pressures were different between the four diet groups, with meat eaters having the highest values and vegans the lowest values. The differences in mean blood pressure between meat eaters and vegans among participants with no self-reported hypertension were 4.2 and 2.6 mmHg systolic and 2.8 and 1.7 mmHg diastolic for men and women, respectively.

The authors concluded that vegans have a lower prevalence of hypertension and lower systolic and diastolic blood pressures than meat eaters, largely because of differences in body mass index. So get your skinny on, get your Plant-Based Solution in gear, and enjoy the lower weight and blood pressure that should follow.

Plant Rant

When it comes to the dietary management or reversal of disease, there is a huge database to recommend the Plant-Based Solution. The data is just too strong to hear much pushback from other diet camps. The only dietary pattern that gets similar accolades is the DASH (Dietary Approach to Stop Hypertension) diet, often rated number one overall. It is interesting that the research group providing guidance to the DASH diet program intended it to be a vegetarian study, funded by the National Institutes of Health (NIH). Yet the NIH believed that acceptance by patients might be higher for an omnivorous dietary pattern, rather than a vegetarian one, and thus removed the study arm that was totally plant-based. I do not doubt that if the scientists were to repeat the study with a plant-based cohort, there would be an even more powerful diet than the DASH diet. The winner would be the Plant-Based Solution, and you do not need to wait. Start that solution today.

THE PLANT-BASED PLAN **How to Eat Out**

You can plan for success eating in a restaurant locally or around the world with just a little effort. You can search websites like Happy Cow and Veg Dining for grocers and eateries around the world that feature healthier choices. If you are traveling, I recommend you print some of the results you found before you travel so you do not need to depend on finding Wi-Fi to look choices up. Packing a few staples like a nut butter and a few healthy food bars might get you through a pinch in an airport or small town. Salads and side dishes are always a good choice. Finally, calling ahead to alert a chef of your vegan diet is appreciated and often results in amazing presentations of plant-based meals.

When you are invited to a meal at the home of meat-eating friends or family members (it's going to happen eventually), offer to contribute a vegan dish (see the recipes in chapter 15). That way, you'll know there will be a dish for you to enjoy, and your friends and family will get to taste some delicious vegan food and learn about why you switched to a healthy and humane diet. But don't be pushy about it. Finally, eat a healthy snack or meal before the gathering so you are not "hangry" over the limited vegan delights.

6

Hello Plants,
Goodbye Cholesterol

Repeat after me, "Cholesterol matters, cholesterol matters." There may be confusion in the media about how cholesterol is "no longer a target" for disease prevention, but poppycock. Over the years, I have seen so many patients suffer major heart attacks, and the only abnormality even after an advanced evaluation was an elevated total and elevated LDL (low-density lipoprotein) cholesterol, an elevated LDL cholesterol particle number (an advanced measure of LDL cholesterol), or perhaps a low HDL (high-density lipoprotein) cholesterol. I would add that an elevated Lipoprotein(a), or Lp(a), cholesterol level is particularly common in families and should be a number you know. You might read that butter is back, meat is a treat, coconut oil is the new kale, high cholesterol is good for you, your brain needs lots and lots of fats, and . . . STOP! This is not science but rather media hype that we have been hearing more and more about.

After intense discussion and debate, the USDA's *2015–2020 Dietary Guidelines for Americans* made it crystal clear when it stated that "people should eat as little dietary cholesterol as possible. In general, foods that are higher in dietary cholesterol, such as fatty meats and high-fat dairy products, are also higher in saturated fats (which should be limited to 10 percent of total calories per day). The primary healthy eating style described in the Dietary Guidelines is limited in saturated fats and thus, dietary cholesterol (about 100–300 mg across the various calorie levels)."[1] Plants have *no* cholesterol. Only animal products have cholesterol. Adopting the Plant-Based Solution is a proven way to lower or eliminate your dietary cholesterol load and at the same time decrease foods richest in saturated fats, like cheese, chicken, meats, and eggs.

Some plant-based foods, while free of cholesterol, are high in saturated fats. None is higher than coconut oil. Coconut oil is not a whole food because it has been processed to remove the water and meat. It is left with a whopping 92 percent of calories from saturated fat. There is no data that coconut oil is good or even safe for heart arteries. (Other coconut-based foods such as milk, yogurt, or sugar are not 100 percent fat and may be acceptable for many people.) Even olive oil is a highly processed food that may have 15–20 percent of calories from saturated fat. Oils are not WFPB but are processed, and important nutrients are ripped out. All the fiber and minerals are gone. Poof! Beware of them and the hype around them.

Cholesterol by the Numbers

	Total Cholesterol	HDL Cholesterol	LDL Cholesterol	Triglycerides
Good	Less than 200	40 or higher	Less than 100	Less than 149
Borderline	200–239	n/a	130–159	150–199
High	240 or higher	n/a	160 or higher	200 or higher
Low	n/a	Less than 40	n/a	n/a

CASE STUDY

Cholesterol and Thirty Days of the Plant-Based Solution

Adam is a lovable guy with a huge following in the business community. His giant smile attracts many to him on social media, and he was known for his posts calling his friends to meet for a late-night food orgy centered on burgers and bacon. He was the most meat-oriented person I had ever met, and I have little doubt he had bacon-scented deodorant and a full-body bacon suit to wear on Halloween.

I was pleased, therefore, when he texted me to say he wanted to try a change, maybe for just thirty days. Then in his late forties, he felt his diet high in processed foods, meat, and fats could not work long term, even though he felt okay. The fact that he ate almost every meal out made it a bit more challenging, but he said he was up to a thirty-day immersion into the Plant-Based Solution. I was stoked.

To document his status at baseline, I arranged advanced labs of his blood and urine. On the first of the month, he was ready to go. I admired his energy and enthusiasm to do this right. He switched out eggs and bacon for oatmeal and fruit. Lunch became soups and vegetable plates. Dinner might be baked potatoes, stir-fries with tofu, or a rare plant-based frozen meal. He posted pictures on social media of our grocery tours where I showed him hundreds of plant-based options. He actually shunned the processed meat substitutes and wanted to concentrate on whole foods.

Adam pretty much stuck to the program for the entire month. He noticed energy, regular bowel frequency with ease, and greater brain clarity. He had never eaten so many fruits and vegetables in his life as in those thirty days. After a month, I repeated his laboratory testing, unsure whether enough time had passed to see changes. However, there were important improvements already: His high-sensitivity C-reactive protein, a measure of dangerous inflammation, fell dramatically from 6.1 mg/l to 0.7, back to the normal range. His body was no longer being irritated by his food choices. A urine test called the MACR, or microalbumin-to-creatinine ratio, fell from 8.5 (a high level, indicating protein was leaking from damaged arteries into his kidneys) to undetectable, indicating a major healing process. Finally, his total cholesterol fell from 224 mg/dl to 196, his LDL cholesterol from 142 to 115, and his LDL particle number (an ideal level being <1,000 mg/dl) from 1,714 mg/dl to 1,474. These improvements lowered his calculated risk of heart attack and stroke significantly and all in just thirty days!

Adam is continuing his journey mixing some of the older habits with many of his new ones. He is single and finds that dating plant-based women keeps him focused. Whatever works, because he is healthier and happier too! ■

Study In-Depth: Cholesterol Medication Versus a Plant-Based Diet

Could a plant-based diet loaded with foods known to lower cholesterol ever compare to a prescription cholesterol-lowering statin medication to control your cholesterol? That is exactly the question asked in a carefully done study published in a prestigious medical research journal.[2]

Forty-six healthy adults with high cholesterol levels (twenty-five men and twenty-one postmenopausal women) were randomly assigned to undergo one of three interventions on an outpatient basis for one month: (1) a diet very low in saturated fat, based on milled whole-wheat cereals and low-fat dairy foods (the non-vegan control group); (2) the same diet plus the powerful cholesterol-lowering medication Mevacor (lovastatin); or (3) a diet high in plant sterols via supplements, soy protein, plant-based fiber, and almonds, all known to lower cholesterol (the "dietary portfolio" group).

The study went on for four weeks. The non-vegan control group, the Mevacor statin group, and the dietary portfolio group all had decreases in LDL ("bad") cholesterol of 8 percent, 31 percent, and 29 percent, respectively. Reductions in the C-reactive protein, a measure of dangerous inflammation, were 10 percent for the control group, 33 percent for the Mevacor group, and 28 percent for the dietary portfolio group. There were no significant differences in efficacy between the Mevacor statin and dietary portfolio treatments even though the dietary portfolio group was not using any prescription medication. That is amazing.

Five Tips for Lowering Your Cholesterol

1. Begin with a *WFPB diet low in salt, oils, fats, and added sugars,* rich in fruits and vegetables.

2. *Take 2 grams of plant stanols daily.* Plant stanols block cholesterol absorption in the GI tract and can be found in the supplement section of natural grocery stores.

3. *Eat about two dozen or 30 grams of almonds a day.* Almonds are rich in minerals, vitamin E, and fiber. Try substituting margarine or peanut butter with almond butter spread on whole-grain breads (but be careful with the amount if you are trying to lose weight).

4. *Aim for 20 grams of soluble fiber a day,* which binds cholesterol in the gut. Two big bowls of oatmeal, lentils, chickpeas, barley, or beans a day, whether alone or added to soups or salads, will meet this goal. Five servings of fruits and vegetables can add half of the target amount of soluble fiber.

5. Finally, soy is high in fiber, low in saturated fat, and a good complete protein source. *The goal is 50 grams of soy a day.* Organic soy milk, tofu, and edamame are good choices. Soy nuts can be a good snack or added to salads, but buy organic and unsalted.

My patients who embraced this diet to lower their cholesterol have seen good results and enjoyed the challenge of fitting these special foods in daily. As always, inch by inch it is a cinch, so go slow.

Science Corner: Proven Cholesterol-Lowering Effects of the Plant-Based Solution

There has been great interest in diet and cholesterol management for a variety of reasons: Heart disease is so common and serious; the medications used have been quite expensive in the past and the new ones

(PCSK9 inhibitors) are even more expensive; and some people encounter side effects (muscle aches and weakness, memory loss, blood sugar elevation) on statin medication. If lowering your cholesterol is a goal you want to achieve naturally, the following studies will be important to you.

Data from the EPIC-Oxford study is important to understand. Researchers in the United Kingdom looked at a sample of over 424 meat eaters, 425 fish eaters, 423 vegetarians, and 422 vegans matched for sex and age.[3] Vegans had the lowest body mass index, the highest intakes of polyunsaturated fat, and the lowest intake of saturated fat. Vegans had the lowest serum concentrations of total and non-HDL cholesterol and apolipoprotein B (ApoB)—all bad cholesterol fractions that you want to be low. The authors concluded that total cholesterol concentrations were lower in vegans compared with meat eaters, fish eaters, and vegetarians. Vegans were also on average thinner, as eating a WFPB diet has multiple benefits.

Some criticize studies like the EPIC-Oxford analysis because while it observed differences in groups—in this case a much lower cholesterol in vegans—it is not a randomized trial comparing two diets. There is one study that fits that bill and may inspire you to choose a WFPB diet to lower your cholesterol.

As I mentioned in chapter 3, Dr. Neal Barnard approached the insurance company GEICO about doing a study of plant-based nutrition for its employees.[4] It was set up as a randomized study in the workplace. Employees from ten sites were randomized to either follow a low-fat vegan diet, with weekly group support and work cafeteria options available, or make no diet changes for eighteen weeks. At intervention sites with cafeterias, low-fat vegan menu options, such as oatmeal, minestrone, lentil soup, and veggie burgers, were among the daily offerings. The low-fat vegan menu options were highlighted in the cafeteria, but the daily vegan options varied depending on the individual cafeterias. All the study subjects were either overweight or had a diagnosis of type 2 diabetes mellitus. Measurements were made before and after the study period.

At the end of eighteen weeks, weight fell only in the vegan group, on average seven pounds. Total and LDL cholesterol fell 8.0 and

8.1 mg/dl in the intervention group and 0.01 and 0.9 mg/dl in the control group. This difference was significant, and clinically would be important. Additional benefits were lower blood pressure and blood-sugar measurements at the end of the study period. This randomized study shows the power of the effects of a low-fat WFPB diet on cholesterol levels.

Another piece of evidence is a recent analysis comparing followers of a vegan diet to similar-aged omnivores. Their cholesterol levels were the main focus of the study.[5] Compared to the omnivores, the vegan subjects had lower total cholesterol, LDL cholesterol, non-HDL cholesterol, and ApoB. Concentration of HDL cholesterol was similar between groups. The study concluded that a vegan diet may have a beneficial effect on the serum lipid profile and cardiovascular protection. Not a bad outcome for eating WFPB diets: less risk for heart disease, the nation's top killer. You can get the same result.

Plant Rant

There is a war going on for your mind and wallet by confusing you about the health aspects of eating foods high in fats, particularly animal saturated fats. For example, a British cardiologist recommends putting butter in coffee and eating full-fat dairy. He even gained international attention with an editorial in the *British Medical Journal* titled "Saturated Fat Is Not the Major Issue."[6] He relies heavily on a meta-analysis in 2010 on the topic of saturated fat and also on a randomized trial examining different versions of a Mediterranean diet on coronary artery disease (CAD) outcomes like heart attack and heart deaths.[7]

I have many issues with doctors who recommend increasing fats like butter in the diet while also telling the public to avoid whole grains. This combination produces a low-carbohydrate, high-fat mix. This is worrisome because the LCHF diet is associated with an increase in all-cause and CAD mortality in large databases.[8] Meat, dairy products, and processed foods high in saturated fat remain the main felon in CAD, with added sugars an obvious accomplice. When you plan your meals, I would strongly recommend you ignore advice from outliers like this particular British physician and remain loyal to the proven Plant-Based Solution.

THE PLANT-BASED PLAN   Have a Smoothie a Day

Increase your daily fruit and vegetable servings by having a smoothie a day. Smoothies don't have to be limited to breakfast. They're great with lunch, as a snack, or for dessert, and they are simple to prepare. I love the NutriBullet blender because it makes one serving at a time, it's powerful, and it's easy to clean, but you can use any blender.

SMOOTHIE

INGREDIENTS

1½   cups liquid (any plant milk or juice or a combination)
1   banana or ½ avocado
1   cup fresh or frozen fruit

OPTIONAL ADD-INS

1   handful of kale or spinach
¼   cup oats
1–2   tablespoons chia seeds or ground flax seeds
1–2   tablespoons nuts or 1 tablespoon nut butter

INSTRUCTIONS

1. Blend all ingredients until smooth.
2. Add more liquid if needed.

7

Grow Plants
Not Cancer Cells

One of the most compelling reasons to adopt the Plant-Based Solution right now is to lower your risk of cancer. Few things scare people more than the fear of a phone call or office visit where they learn that cancer is the diagnosis. No matter how it is diagnosed (biopsy, CT scan, or blood test), cancer is common and frightening.

How common is cancer in the United States? The National Cancer Institute estimates that in 2016 there were 1,685,210 new cases of cancer and that 595,690 people died from the disease.[1] That is like filling the Big House stadium in Ann Arbor, Michigan, which holds over 100,000 people, six times, and no one makes it out alive. That is a lot of loved ones. And that is just in one year.

The most common cancers in 2016, in order of prevalence, were:

1. bladder cancer
2. breast cancer
3. colon and rectal cancer
4. endometrial cancer
5. kidney cancer
6. leukemia
7. liver cancer
8. lung cancer
9. melanoma of the skin
10. non-Hodgkin's lymphoma
11. pancreatic cancer
12. prostate cancer
13. thyroid cancer

Cancer deaths are highest in the United States in African American men. About 15 million to 16 million Americans are living with a cancer diagnosis, and that number is expected to rise to almost 19 million by 2024. Approximately 40 percent of American men and women will be diagnosed with cancer at some point during their lifetime.[2]

The problem is not isolated to the United States. According to the National Cancer Institute, cancer is among the leading causes of death worldwide. In 2012, there were 14 million new cases and 8 million cancer-related deaths worldwide. More than 60 percent of the world's new cancer cases occur in Africa, Asia, and Central and South America; 70 percent of the world's cancer deaths also occur in these regions.[3]

In the United States, the overall cancer death rate has been declining since the early 1990s, and in the most recent National Cancer Institute report, it continued to drop.[4] Nonetheless, hundreds of thousands of people are still dying yearly of cancer, and if nutrition can prevent even a few cases, then information should be taught and shared everywhere possible. You can lower your risk for cancer, and here is the data to support your journey.

Science Corner: The WHO and Processed Red Meats

The medical world was caught by surprise in October 2015 when an announcement by the International Agency for Research on Cancer (IARC), an agency of the World Health Organization (WHO), known for expertise in analyzing scientific data for health risks, declared that meat acts as a carcinogen.[5] Processed red meats include bacon, pepperoni, bologna, hot dogs, salami, and corned beef, and these foods were found to cause colorectal cancer. Those are strong words. Not maybe or might, but definitely cause cancer. The analysis placed processed red meat as a Group 1 carcinogen similar to diesel fumes and tobacco. These strong determinations shocked many and made headlines worldwide.[6] In case you missed it, the IARC, made up of twenty-two scientists from ten countries, reviewed over 800 studies and ruled that:

- Processed meats like bacon, ham, salami, sausage, and beef jerky are Group 1 carcinogens, the highest risk assigned, which means they cause cancer. The relationship was strongest with colorectal cancer (CRC) and stomach cancer but also existed for other cancers like pancreatic and prostate.

- The risk increases incrementally with the amount of these meats eaten. Each 50 gram portion of processed meat daily increases the risk of colorectal cancer by 18 percent.

- Fresh red meats, like steak and roasts as well as pork and lamb, were considered as probable causes of cancer to humans (Group 2a) with links to colorectal, pancreatic, and prostate cancer.

The IARC report followed similar prior reports like that of the World Cancer Research Fund,[7] which identified the same causation.

The news about processed red meats and cancer made headlines for a few days but was quickly forgotten, at least in hospital cafeterias and wards. There is new research indicating how the recommendations of the IARC could reduce the risk of colorectal cancer if applied widely.[8] Six dietary and lifestyle recommendations (body weight, physical activity, energy density, plant foods, red and processed meat, and alcohol) were examined in terms of their association with CRC incidence over more than seven years of follow-up in 66,920 adults aged fifty to seventy-six with no history of CRC. The analysis indicated that participants meeting one to three preventive recommendations enjoyed a 34 to 45 percent lower CRC incidence than those who followed none of them, while those meeting four to six of the targets experienced a 58 percent lower incidence of CRC. In both men and women, the lowest risk for cancer was achieved by avoiding processed red meats like bacon. I am sure you would like to drop your risk of colon cancer by over 50 percent even if it means changing your diet to a cancer prevention pattern.

The burden of tragedy for CRC in the United States is enormous. In 2014, about 140,000 people were diagnosed with CRC and nearly 50,000 died of this disease.[9] African American men and women experience the highest rates of CRC, as much as 50 percent higher than whites, and should be spreading the word in their communities to eat plants, not bacon and sausage.

Processed Red Meats and Hospital Food

I want you to get as mad as I am. Outraged. You heard it already in an earlier chapter, but let's have a moment of good, old-fashioned anger again. How can hospitals knowingly contribute to cancer by serving foods classified as carcinogens? Hospitals banned smoking after risk of cancer was established. Why have they not committed to tackling cancer prevention in all manners? Is it okay for hospitals to avoid cancer prevention if it might hurt their finances and invite criticism from workers and the public by banning popular foods? Hospitals are now facing an ethical choice regarding the WHO statements on processed red meats. Is it appropriate for a medical center to continue serving hot dogs, sausages, bacon, ham, bologna, and salami? I bring these questions up because as you start your journey on the Plant-Based Solution, you might wonder why Group 1 carcinogens are being served in hospitals. It confuses a lot of people.

Not only is colorectal cancer the third most common cancer diagnosed in the United States each year, but it also causes terrible pain and suffering during therapy. This can include disfiguring surgery, chemotherapy, radiation therapy, and the risk of death. If even a few more deaths yearly are related to hospitals serving processed meats, it is a tragic error.

I went to my main hospital administrators and asked for a meeting to discuss banning processed meats on the principle that medical centers should not cause cancer knowingly. I persisted with emails until I heard a response: "People should have a choice." A choice, like a pack of Lucky Strikes or Marlboros? Asbestos or diesel exhaust fumes? What people do in their own homes or free time is a personal choice, but the food served in hospitals must be held to a higher standard.

According to the American Medical Association, a hospital's ethical responsibility is to make the health-promoting choice the easy choice. Just as doctors (derived from the Latin *docere*, "to teach") are responsible for teaching individual patients about good eating habits, so are the hospital systems for which they work responsible for promoting dietary change. At least one major hospital system has announced a total ban on processed red meats in accord with the WHO data (Kaiser Permanente, discussed in chapter 1). Others must follow suit. If you are ever admitted to a hospital, and I hope you are not, ask for a plant-based meal and see the staff scratch their heads.

Hot Question: Can I Eat Starchy Vegetables and Still Be Healthy?

Do you have to stick to leafy green vegetables like kale to succeed on your journey with the Plant-Based Solution, or can you eat a baked squash, rice, beans, and even white potatoes? Dr. John McDougall, who you read about in chapter 5, is not only a warrior for whole-starch diets, he has led the charge for forty years. With his McDougall Program, he has seen huge success with patients by emphasizing a diet rich in complex carbohydrates from plant-based starches.

Dr. McDougall developed the diet in the early 1970s when he was practicing medicine on a sugar plantation in Hawaii. He observed the health of plantation workers decline as they traded their starch-rich diets of native Asian countries, with lots of rice and potatoes, for new American choices. The second and third generations of immigrant workers experienced new and serious health problems as a result.

He began treating patients with plant-based diets that were also free of vegetable oils (but were rich in common starches, such as corn, rice, oats, barley, potatoes, sweet potatoes, beans, peas, and lentils). Fresh fruit and non-starchy green, orange, and yellow vegetables were also included. Overall, the diet was about 80 percent complex carbohydrates, 12 percent protein, and 8 percent fat. Spices were also used, along with small amounts of salt and sugar.

Dr. McDougall published a study in *Nutrition Journal* that showed the effects of one week of following the program. After seven days, there was an average weight loss of three pounds. And even though most blood pressure and diabetic medications were reduced or eliminated on the first day, systolic blood pressure fell 8 mmHg and blood glucose also dropped. Heart disease risk calculated with a standard formula fell from greater than 7.5 percent over ten years to 5.5 percent.

Whether it is corn and yucca among Native Americans, potatoes in South America, millet in Africa, barley in the Middle East, rice in Asia, or sorghum in East Africa, human civilization has been powered by starch throughout history. The chronic afflictions of heart attacks, type 2 diabetes, obesity, and dementia, which plague our society, were all rare in these native populations. In Okinawa, Japan, where people have lived longest in the world, their traditional diet was at least 80 percent from carbohydrates, most of which were varieties of sweet potatoes.

For more information and a little bit of humor, you can download a free picture book that Dr. McDougall created, *Food Poisoning: How to Cure It by Eating Beans, Corn, Pasta, Potatoes, Rice, Etc.*

Study In-Depth: Shrinking Prostate Cancer with Plants

Dr. Dean Ornish, who revolutionized "lifestyle medicine" for heart health, did not limit his research on a plant-based lifestyle program to heart disease. He planned and executed experiments in men with prostate cancer who had been chosen for "watchful waiting"—not to be treated with drugs or surgery—for reasons unrelated to Ornish's study. This was done with the head of urology at the University of California's San Francisco School of Medicine, Dr. Peter Carroll. Dr. Ornish identified ninety-three men who had prostate cancer and were being observed without surgery or radiation therapy.[10] The men were randomized into a conventional treatment group that followed up with their urologists as planned and a second group that enrolled in the Ornish Lifestyle Medicine Program—a plant-based diet without added oils or fats (no nuts, seeds, avocados, or oils while minimizing sugar and refined carbs) that included stress management with yoga and meditation, walking for exercise, and social support.

At the end of a year, none in the lifestyle group had progressed to needing additional treatment like surgery or radiation, but six of the control patients did need such surgery for the growth of their tumor. The serum PSA level, a tumor marker, fell by 4 percent in the lifestyle group while it increased by 6 percent in the control group.

The researchers took blood from both groups and dropped it on prostate cancer cells growing in Petri dishes. The growth of the cancer cells was inhibited almost eight times as often in the lifestyle group versus the control group! This is like the blood becoming a form of chemotherapy itself when it is rich in plant-based foods without dairy and added fats. The more the subjects fully adhered to the program, the more their blood killed cancer cells! What a great reason to learn to love broccoli. In fact, the cruciferous vegetable family, which includes broccoli, cauliflower, greens, mustards, and wasabi, is one of the most potent food groups you can choose to impact prostate cancer cell growth.

I have cared for hundreds of men with prostate cancer since this research study was published, and not one had heard from their medical team that lifestyle habits could help shrink their cancer. Maybe you are one of these men or know one of them. I routinely tell them to search online for Dr. Ornish and prostate cancer, and they will find all they need to read to implement the changes. The same study has not been done with breast cancer because it is not standard to advise a group of women with biopsy-proven cancer to simply watch their disease. However, there are many similarities in the response of breast cancer cells and prostate cancer cells, and it would be wise to inform a woman about the results of the Ornish prostate cancer study so she can make an informed decision.

Feeding the Prostate Healthy Choices

I met Jeff over a decade ago when he was referred by his doctor for management of his cholesterol. He was a friendly man from the start but quite busy in a high-pressure law firm as a partner trying cases. During the course of working with him on lifestyle measures to manage his cholesterol, including educating him about the ability of plant-based diets to lower his cholesterol levels, he was diagnosed with prostate cancer and was recommended to have radiation therapy. He recovered, and on the next visit we discussed his options.

The data from Dr. Ornish's clinical trial on prostate cancer had just been published, and I reviewed it with Jeff. He had a great zest for life, a beautiful wife, children, and grandchildren. He also loved golf and decided if changes could improve his odds of remaining cancer-free for decades ahead, he was in. He moved his diet more and more to the Plant-Based Solution and seemed to enjoy the empowerment it gave him to know that three times a day at least he was voting for life and health with his fork and spoon.

Now, a dozen years later, every urology checkup is good news while he consistently gets good cardiology reports from me too. The power of the Plant-Based Solution to promote optimal blood pressure, blood cholesterol, blood sugar, body weight, heart health, cancer prevention, and as you will see, brain health and other benefits, is truly breathtaking. At the same time, he is making the world a cleaner and safer place for those grandchildren he loves so much. Good work, Jeff, health hero! ■

Science Corner: Studies Support the Plant-Based Solution for Cancer Prevention

You might be wondering if the Plant-Based Solution can prevent the development of prostate cancer in the first place. The familiar Adventist Health Study studied a large group of 26,346 male participants for this risk.[11] In total, 1,079 incident prostate cancer cases were identified. About 8 percent of the study population reported adherence to the vegan diet. Vegan diets showed a statistically significant protective association with prostate cancer risk, reducing it by about 35 percent. Vegan diets were protective in both whites and blacks, an important finding, as the incidence of prostate cancer in African Americans is the highest of all demographic groups. The authors concluded that vegan diets may confer a lower risk of prostate cancer.

What happens to the risk of CRC when adopting a vegetarian dietary pattern? The Adventist Health Study looked at the relationship between dietary pattern and risk of CRC in over 77,000 participants.[12] In a follow-up over seven years, about 500 new cases of CRC were diagnosed. The risk of CRC was reduced by over 20 to 30 percent in vegetarians versus non-vegetarians. As there are around 130,000 new cases of CRC diagnosed yearly in the United States alone, this is tens of thousands of cases of a tragic diagnosis that might be avoided with the Plant-Based Solution.

Another group of subjects have been followed prospectively in the United Kingdom. Their dietary pattern and risk for overall cancer rates have been examined in detail and published in a peer-reviewed medical journal.[13] Over 61,000 British citizens were studied, including 32,491 meat eaters, 8,612 fish eaters, and 20,544 vegetarians (including 2,246 vegans). Cancer incidence was followed through nationwide cancer registries. After an average follow-up of fifteen years, there were 4,998 cancers: 3,275 in meat eaters (10 percent), 520 in fish eaters (6 percent), and 1,203 in vegetarians (6 percent). Stomach cancer was reduced by over 60 percent in vegetarians. Cancers of the lymphoid and hematopoietic tissues like leukemia were reduced by over 35 percent in vegetarians. Multiple myeloma, a cancer of the bone marrow, was reduced by almost 80 percent in vegetarians. Overall, the combined data from the Adventist and the British studies, with over 130,000 subjects studied and followed for years, makes the case that we could empty oncology wards and chemotherapy centers by teaching and implementing simple strategies to favor plants over animals. Share this information with your friends and loved ones.

Cruciferous Vegetables Are Crucial in Cancer Prevention

If you had to put your emphasis on only a single plant-based food group to impact your risk of developing cancer or your recovery from cancer, you would want to concentrate on the brassica family of cruciferous vegetables. These vegetables include broccoli, kale, bok choy, mustard greens, cauliflower, wasabi mustards, cabbage, arugula, watercress, and turnips. Many studies show that the higher the intake of these foods, the lower the risk of cancers.[14] There is a beneficial chemical called sulforaphane that can be produced by eating these foods. Sulforaphane leads to an increase in the production of protective antioxidants via a pathway called nrf2.

The trick to getting the most sulforaphane from your cruciferous vegetables is to chew them. Cruciferous vegetables are like a "glow stick" because before you break them open by chewing, two chemicals are kept apart. The enzyme called myrosinase is separated from the precursor of sulforaphane called glucophoranin. These are big words but with big benefits. When these foods are chewed and the cell walls broken down, the precursor and the enzyme mix together producing the sulforaphane, and then the nrf2 pathway gets activated.

How to Get the Glow Stick Effect

If you cook your cruciferous vegetables heavily before chewing them, the delicate myrosinase enzyme may be damaged and unable to activate the sulforaphane. You still get lots of fiber and other nutrients but less of the cancer-fighting properties of cruciferous vegetables. There are several strategies to activate the myrosinase enzyme during cooking to maximize the antioxidant benefits:

- Chop the vegetables and let them sit before cooking. This mimics chewing and allows the chemical reaction to occur outside the body before the heat is applied. After fifteen to thirty minutes, you can cook them any way you prefer.

- Add a few pieces of the raw vegetable, like a few broccoli florets, into the bigger bowl of cooked vegetable and mix them. The raw pieces still have the active myrosinase enzyme to spark the health reaction.

- Sprinkle dried mustard powder on the bowl of cooked vegetables. Mustard is part of the brassica family and has the myrosinase enzyme retained. It adds a distinct flavor with a bit of a bite that is quite tasteful, and when you sprinkle it on, you ignite the "glow stick" reaction.

Cruciferous vegetables have been called "frugal chemoprevention" against cancer and are one form of natural protection you want to use regularly.[15]

Plant Rant

There are so many studies supporting the powerful role of the Plant-Based Solution on the prevention and treatment of cancer that this should be common knowledge and standard medical advice. In most of the studies, the vegan dietary pattern was superior to other versions of a vegetarian diet. Try to get five, ten, or even more servings of fruits and vegetables, whole grains, and legumes into your daily routine. Add a variety of types and colors to gain all the benefits. Emphasize cruciferous vegetables served to maximize sulforaphane production.

You may still wonder about all the talk of high-profile diets featuring animal products: the message that butter is back; that a low-carb, high-fat, meat-centric diet is good for you or necessary for your hormones or brain; that full-fat dairy, like adding cheese to your diet, as some of my colleagues now recommend, is healthy. And what about hospitals serving processed red meats known to be carcinogens? You know the real data now, and you know that the lowest risk of developing cancer for you and your family is by sticking to the science of the Plant-Based Solution.

THE PLANT-BASED PLAN **Make Vegetable Broth**

You will see in my recipes in chapter 15 that I often use vegetable broth when cooking. You can make a batch and freeze it in 1- to 2-cup portions or in ice-cube trays. Then, just take out a 1- or 2-cup portion for a recipe or pop out one or two cubes when you need a little broth for sautéing. This is an easy way to replace the oil and reduce your daily fat intake without sacrificing flavor. Wine, vinegar, or water can also be used.

VEGETABLE BROTH

INGREDIENTS

2–3 carrots, chopped

1 onion, chopped

2 stalks celery, chopped

Several sprigs fresh parsley

Bay leaf

OPTIONAL ADD-INS

A few tablespoons of brown lentils

A handful of any type of mushrooms, chopped

A few garlic cloves, minced

A few sun-dried tomatoes, chopped

Springs of fresh thyme

1 tablespoon whole peppercorns

INSTRUCTIONS

1. Combine the carrots, onion, celery, parsley, and bay leaf in a large stockpot filled with water.
2. Toss in optional add-ins.
3. Bring to boil, and gently simmer uncovered for 2 to 3 hours.
4. Strain, cool, and refrigerate or freeze.

8

Beans Not Butter
for Better Brains

Ever forget your keys? Where your car is parked? Who you were about to call? The fear of losing memory and the loss of control over other functions of the brain and neurologic system is a worry that many of my patients have expressed. Our brain makes us human and gives us the unique personality and skills we each have. Preserving brain and neurological function by a mindful dietary pattern emphasizing plants over animals is worthy of examination. The fact that a cauliflower looks a lot like a brain does not prove the point that a plant-based diet is the best pattern for brain health. But as you will see, it may not be a coincidence either.

Multiple Sclerosis

If you worry about your brain, then you need to know about a diet that has been studied for a common neurological disease, multiple sclerosis, or MS. MS is an autoimmune and inflammatory disease of the nervous system that can lead to severely disabling manifestations. A therapy for MS using a predominantly plant-based diet has been studied in patients followed for decades at a major university neurology clinic. This diet, constructed to be low in fat, is known as the Swank diet and is an important milestone.[1]

Roy Swank, MD, served as professor of neurology at the Oregon Health & Science University and passed away in 2008 at age ninety-nine. He theorized decades ago that the increased incidence of MS in northern countries might be due to decreased plant-based foods and increased animal foods. Others have implicated differences in sunshine and vitamin D production, but Swank thought otherwise. In addition, he noticed that in Norway, people who lived in fishing communities were eight times less likely to develop MS than those who lived in the mountains where meat was the main dietary component. According to Julie Stachowiak, PhD, "Swank noted that after eating a high-fat meal, a person's blood cells could clump together and be able to block circulation in capillaries. He hypothesized that these clumps were blocking the tiny blood vessels in the blood-brain barrier and leading to inflammation and lesions in the central nervous system. His theory was that if you cut out the fat (saturated fat), you eliminate the clumps of blood cells." No more clumping might mean no more blockages and no more inflammation, which could mean no more MS lesions.[2]

Professor Swank embarked on studying a diet plan that was low in saturated fats from dairy and meat while high in fruits and vegetables. It was not a vegan diet, though red meat was not permitted in the first year of care. Swank reported a decrease in the frequency and severity of MS attacks. He continued to add patients and followed up with them over thirty-four years of this nutritional treatment,[3] a remarkable length of time for a study! The greatest benefit was seen in those who began the diet early in their MS course. After deaths from non-MS causes were excluded, a startling 95 percent survived and remained physically active. The patients who increased their saturated fat intake over time had a striking increase in average disability and death. Swank later tracked down patients on his diet after fifty years and reported on thirteen of them who continued to do well and had youthful appearances.[4] He concluded that MS was probably due in part to saturated fat.

The actual mechanisms of the Swank diet on ameliorating the symptoms of MS are unknown, but theories have been proposed.[5] Whatever the exact mechanism, the Swank diet has been hailed as an effective, if not *the* most effective, treatment in the literature.[6] A shortcoming of the work in MS patients pioneered by Dr. Swank was the absence of brain MRI data on his patients, as the technique was not available when his studies began.

Recently Dr. John McDougall teamed up with the Department of Neurology of the same university Dr. Swank served at for years.[7] Patients were monitored on a diet that had either 15 percent of calories from fat or 40 percent from fat. Compliance was high, and there was far more weight loss and decline in blood cholesterol measurements in the lower-fat cohort. Although it was hoped that brain MRI studies done before the diet and after a year on the diet would show clear improvements, the MRI results at the end of the year did not differ significantly. Overall, the study group was probably too small and the study time period too short to provide any imaging conclusions; thus, further work will be needed. While we don't yet know how saturated fat harms the brain in patients with MS, thanks to Swank's comprehensive research we do know that a plant-based diet helps MS in some manner.

CASE STUDY
Taming MS with Plants

I met Sarah because of some skipped and racing heartbeats she was experiencing now and then. After an evaluation that showed a healthy heart and normal laboratory studies, she was able to eliminate the problem by reducing her caffeine intake and using some supplemental magnesium at night as a sleep aid.

What was more interesting about Sarah was that she also had MS. She was diagnosed in 2001, about twelve years before I met her. She had been experiencing some changes in her vision. She also felt tingling in her left leg and arm, which she imagined was a pinched nerve, perhaps from an old high-school volleyball injury. When she began to feel some burning in her leg and an overall fatigue, she knew she needed an evaluation. Her primary care doctor ran routine testing that was unrevealing, but a neurologist performed a battery of tests and imaging that was consistent with the diagnosis of MS—a diagnosis she did not want to hear at age forty-four.

A family member residing on the West Coast was familiar with the work of Dr. Swank. He suggested to Sarah that she read his book, *The Multiple Sclerosis Diet Book*, and study his work. At the time, Dr.

Swank was still alive, and Sarah decided to travel from Michigan and meet him in his clinic. She was impressed with his conviction that she could control the disease by adopting the diet he had prescribed to patients for decades. She not only adopted the very low saturated fat guideline, she decided to opt out of all animal products as much as she could and develop skills to create delicious plant-based meals for her and her family.

She is convinced her decision paid off. Within six months of changing her diet she felt her energy was back to normal and the tingling and burning had resolved. She continued to follow up with her local neurologist, who concurred with her stability over the years as he monitored the MS. She never was put on medications for the MS. She does not need any assistance in her daily activities of caring for a new grandchild. She has not needed a walker or wheelchair. She is also no longer having palpitations. ■

Stroke

Have you ever known anyone who had a stroke? Do you have a fear of a stroke? Some strokes are minor, but a major stroke can be life altering and lead to serious disabilities. The Adventist Health Study looked twice at the effect of a vegan diet and stroke.[8] One study was called the Adventist Mortality Study (looking at deaths), and one was the more recent Adventist Health Study analysis. Members of the Seventh-day Adventist community who followed a vegan diet by consuming only plant-based foods had between a 7 and 35 percent lower rate of cerebrovascular disease (stroke syndromes) than the meat-eating omnivores in the study.

There are many possible reasons why this might be, such as the lower blood pressure, lower cholesterol, and reduced rate of type 2 diabetes in vegans. Obesity is also less frequent in vegans, and the associated sleep apnea, atrial fibrillation, and possible emboli (clots traveling from the heart to brain) may be reduced by following a WFPB diet. Whatever the exact reasons, the lower stroke risk in the Adventist vegan groups is important data.

Alzheimer's Disease

Alzheimer's disease affects in excess of 5 million Americans, and it is expected to triple in frequency in coming decades. It is likely something you fear and want to avoid. Although there are several factors known to contribute to the risk of developing Alzheimer's disease—including family history, head trauma, hypertension, obesity, diabetes, and high cholesterol—the possibility that diet plays a role has been considered. Plant-based diets deserve some serious consideration as a preventive strategy.

Over twenty years ago, an early phase of the Adventist Health Study examined the relationship between dementia and diets rich in animal products.[9] The study reported on 272 study subjects living in California who were "matched" for age, sex, and zip code. All subjects were enrolled in the Adventist Health Study, so they had filled out extensive dietary questionnaires. The people who ate meat (including poultry and fish) were more than twice as likely to become demented as their vegetarian counterparts. Not only was dementia less common in those who did not eat meat, but its onset in those who did develop it tended to be delayed. It is certainly better to develop dementia late in life as opposed to early, yet never developing it is the goal.

If you are wondering why the Plant-Based Solution might protect the brain from dementia, there are two theories. One relates to eating greens and their content of folate (notice *folate*, a B vitamin, and *foliage*, or greens, share a common root). Folate is naturally found in whole foods. Folic acid, which is used to supplement foods like cereals, is synthetic.

In the first theory, recall from chapter 5 a process in the body called methylation, which regulates homocysteine, an amino acid that can cause arteries feeding the brain to malfunction. Bad arteries can lead to "bad" brains, and vascular dementia is a major cause of dementia. Better arteries from plant-based diets rich in folate may ward off dementia. Methylation is involved in controlling the activity of genes and the proteins that they control. A common genetic defect in methylation, called a MTHFR defect, is found in as many as 50 percent of people and is severe in perhaps 10 percent. The genetic defect in methylation can lead to cells not functioning normally and to the accumulation of homocysteine. You can ask your doctor for blood tests that determine both the status of the MTHFR gene inheritance and homocysteine levels in the blood to guide the replacement of folate not only with food-based folate but with additional B12 and B6 vitamins too, which are involved in methylation.

The second theory relates to another gene, the ApoE gene. We inherit one ApoE gene from each parent. There are three ApoE gene types called E2, E3, and E4. The ideal inheritance is called ApoE3/3, which means each parent gives the favored ApoE3 gene and represents a low risk of cardiovascular disease and dementia. However, many people inherit one or two ApoE4 genes, with the combination ApoE4/4 (both parents gave an ApoE4 gene) raising the risks of both cardiovascular disease and dementia. A simple blood test can determine this. In individuals with one or two ApoE4 genes, diets high in saturated fats are more likely to raise cholesterol and injure arteries. Diets low in saturated fat are recommended for this group to protect the brain and heart.

If you follow the Plant-Based Solution by eating a healthy WFPB diet, it will be naturally low in saturated fats (because it will omit cheeses, full-fat dairy, chicken, red meats, and other common sources of saturated fats). Whether you know your ApoE status or not, the Plant-Based Solution will be a brain-friendly choice for this reason.

Test Your Brain Health

Ask your doctor for the following tests that assess whether you are at higher risk for stroke, heart disease, and dementia.

MTHFR: This mouthful stands for methyl tetrahydrofolate reductase, an enzyme that is in every cell in the body and required for proper metabolism. The enzyme activity is determined by what genes we inherit from our parents. Each of our parents may donate a normal gene, so we get the normal, or "wild," type. If one parent donates a normal gene and one an altered gene, this enzyme and the process of controlling our metabolism (called methylation) work at only 40 to 50 percent efficiency. Finally, if both parents donate an altered gene, we are homozygous for the MTHFR gene, and we may methylate, or control our metabolism, at only 10 percent the normal efficiency. All of this can be assessed by a simple blood test and will reveal whether we are at higher risk for heart disease.

Homocysteine levels: Homocysteine is an amino acid that cycles with its pal methionine in the same methylation cycle in which the MTHFR enzyme is active. If we inherit altered MTHFR genes, our homocysteine level may rise and cause arteries to malfunction and increase the risk of stroke. This is another lab test. Elevated levels can be corrected with B complex vitamins.

ApoE gene blood test: This blood test assesses whether your parents donated normal versions of the gene called ApoE or an altered one. The most normal is when both parents donate the ApoE3 copy, which is ApoE3/3. This is the lowest risk for stroke, heart attack, and Alzheimer's. More concerning is if you inherit one or two copies of ApoE4, thereby being ApoE4/4. This increases the risk of stroke, heart attack, and dementia. It also suggests the need to decrease saturated fats in the diet (something we all should be doing) and limit alcohol intake.

Seven Guidelines to Prevent Alzheimer's Disease

By now you know I admire the work of Dr. Neal Barnard of the Physicians Committee for Responsible Medicine. Along with co-authors, he has developed guidelines to prevent Alzheimer's disease using diet and lifestyle based on available scientific studies.[10] These are:

1. Minimize your intake of saturated fats and trans fats by avoiding dairy products, meats, and certain oils (coconut and palm oils).

2. Eat vegetables, legumes (beans, peas, and lentils), fruits, and whole grains in place of meats and dairy products as primary staples of the diet.

3. Get your vitamin E from seeds, nuts, green leafy vegetables, and whole grains; vitamin E is a preferred antioxidant for brain health.

4. Consume a source of vitamin B12 daily. Blood levels of vitamin B12 should be checked regularly.

5. Avoid iron and copper in over-the-counter supplements if a multivitamin is being used.

6. Consider minimizing exposure to aluminum by choosing cookware, antacids, baking powder, and other products that are free of added aluminum.

7. Schedule aerobic exercise for at least forty minutes three times per week. Brisk walking can suffice.

Science Corner: Smile but Don't Say Cheese

If you follow a WFPB diet, will you feel happier and less depressed? Wouldn't that be a nice side effect of eating healthier? A study of thirty-nine omnivores suggests this may be true, perhaps through a healthier GI track (the microbiome).[11] The subjects were fed one of three meal patterns: (1) meat, fish, and poultry as an omnivorous diet; (2) a diet with fish three to four times a week but no meat or poultry; or (3) a vegetarian diet free of meat, fish, and dairy. At baseline and at the end of two weeks, assessments of mood states as well as measures of stress, anxiety, and depression were performed. After the study period, the vegetarian group demonstrated several measures of mood scores not seen in the other diets.

While it is not entirely certain why these changes might occur, the authors described differences in dietary fatty acids, like lower levels of arachidonic acid, an inflammatory compound, in the vegetarian group. Don't worry, be happy, go vegan.

Parkinson's Disease

Over a decade ago a hypothesis was presented that plant-based diets may reduce the risk of developing Parkinson's disease.[12] Studies suggested diets higher in animal fat were associated with a higher risk of Parkinson's disease while fat derived from plants, like avocados, did not raise the risk. Therefore, WFPB diets, free of animal fats, offered a hopeful approach.

A bizarre twist on this hypothesis was published about the same time that related to bowel frequency. The study, which analyzed more than 6,700 men free of Parkinson's disease as to their bowel frequency and then followed them for twenty-four years, suggested a link.[13] Subjects with the lowest bowel movement frequency (less than one a day) had four to five times the risk of Parkinson's disease compared to the group with the highest frequency of bowel movements (more than two a day). Even after adjusting for exercise, laxatives, and servings of fruits and vegetables per day, the risk of infrequent bowel movements persisted.

Vegans are good at a lot of things, but they are very good at bowel movement frequency.[14] Compared to omnivores, a study of over 20,000 subjects identified the vegan diet as an independent factor with higher bowel movement frequency. While it is premature to state that eating a WFPB diet is a proven path to prevent or reverse Parkinson's disease, the data is mounting, and the interest in using the nutrients in fruits and vegetables for neuroprotection is growing.[15]

Plant Rant

Do you think most patients with multiple sclerosis ever hear about the results of the Swank diet? Are they ever told that there is fifty years of data on a diet plan that may calm their disease and improve their clinical course? As in heart disease and cancer therapy, full disclosure of the impact of dietary interventions on disease course and prognosis is rarely presented. This is a huge omission and an ethical concern. The times are changing slowly but for the positive, and there is hope that lectures will more routinely incorporate the power of the Plant-Based Solution in medical education. Protect your brain by spending time in your garden, farmers markets, and produce aisles.

THE PLANT-BASED PLAN Prepare Beans and Grains for the Week

One way to save time during the week is to make one big batch of brown rice or quinoa and a big batch of beans that you can eat all week. Sure, you can buy canned beans, but you may like homemade ones better. Use the precooked beans, rice, and quinoa for the recipes in chapter 15, or add a big spoonful of each to a salad or soup.

Brown Rice: Bring 4 cups of water to a boil. Add 2 cups of rinsed rice. When it reaches a boil, reduce heat, cover, and simmer for 45 minutes, or until rice is cooked through and all the water is absorbed. Turn off heat and let rest for 10 minutes. Fluff with a fork and serve, or allow to cool and then store in the refrigerator or freezer. Makes 4 cups of rice.

Quinoa: Bring 4 cups of water or vegetable broth to a boil. Add 2 cups of rinsed quinoa. Cover, reduce heat to low, and simmer for 15 minutes or until tender and the water is absorbed. Fluff with a fork and serve, or allow to cool and then store in the refrigerator or freezer. Makes 4 cups of quinoa.

Beans: In a large pot, combine 10 cups of water and 3 cups of dried beans, rinsed. Heat to boiling. Remove from heat and cover. Let sit for 1 hour. Simmer partially covered beans for 2 to 4 hours (chickpeas may take 4 hours and smaller beans will be quicker) until soft. Keep an eye on them—you may have to add more water. There is no need to presoak beans. (To save time, consider using a pressure cooker—beans will cook in less than an hour.) Makes 6 cups of beans. Refrigerate (or freeze) in 1½-cup portions, which is roughly the quantity in one 15-ounce can.

9

Grow Plants
Not Autoimmune Diseases

War, what is it good for? You know the answer: absolutely nothing. The same is true when the war is internal in the human body and vital tissues are attacked by our own immune system. This is often called an autoimmune condition, and there are dozens of examples, including perhaps multiple sclerosis, mentioned in the last chapter. Other well-known conditions include systemic lupus erythematosus (SLE), rheumatoid arthritis, psoriasis, and some thyroid diseases.

An estimated 50 million Americans suffer from an autoimmune disease, and the number is rising fast. We often do not understand why the body begins to attack itself and causes the immune cells to activate against the body, but our microbiome, the bacteria we live with inside our colon, may play an important role. Some estimates suggest that there are ten times as many bacteria in our colon as the total number of cells in our entire body, into the trillions and trillions. The bacterial mix can favor a healthy immune response or activate uncontrolled inflammation.

Although not all the pathways between alterations in the microbiome and the activity of the immune system are known, recent studies support the strong connection and the opportunity to alter and treat the autoimmune response by supporting a healthy microbiome.[1] The potential to reset the microbiome toward a more favorable mixture of bacteria is promising, whether by probiotic bacterial strains in food or capsules or by altering the diet to the Plant-Based Solution. Dietary and lifestyle changes provide a powerful path to suppress autoimmune diseases. Healthy gut bacteria can be harmed by antibiotics, a high-fat diet, life stress, endocrine disruptors like the BPA in plastics, and possibly food-based hormones and genetically modified components.

Can WFPB diets really help your microbiome and its input into your immune system? Leafy greens, legumes like lentils, nuts, seeds, fruits, and, for most people, 100 percent whole grains all support a healthy GI population of bacteria. One reason WFPB diets are healthy is that they serve up a rich supply of fiber. Fiber can be food to the good bacteria. Resistant starch found in boiled potatoes, for example, can also be a good supply to repopulate healthy bacteria. Fermented plant-based foods actually have large numbers of healthy bacteria, so fermented vegetables, sauerkraut, and miso are all attractive food choices.

Another reason why WFPB diets can promote a healthy microbiome is that they are naturally low in saturated fat and overall fat content. Diets high in saturated fat may trigger the release of bacterial toxins into the bloodstream.[2] Meat can be loaded with unhealthy bacteria products, hopefully dead, and can also carry with it the antibiotics, hormones, pesticides, and other potential poisons that enter our body and can weaken our immune response.

A WFPB diet itself is associated with less inflammation than animal-based products. The supply of vitamin C, vitamin E, and other nutrients that support wellness and healthy immunity are much richer in plant-based foods. Because plant-based foods are usually free of antibiotic contamination, the opportunity to support a healthy microbiome is maximized.

Organic Versus Conventional: Does It Matter for the Health of Your Family?

Before leaving the topic of the microbiome and WFPB diets, a word on the issue of organic versus conventional produce is in order. There is no question that if the only supply of produce is conventional due to budget constraints or availability, eat the conventional produce. The benefits of eating vegetables and fruits from conventionally grown sources are so abundant that there should be no hesitation in eating them. But what happens if you try to reduce your ingestion of pesticides and other contaminants?

Researchers in Australia studied thirteen volunteers for two weeks.[3] For one week volunteers ate a conventional diet, and for one week they ate a diet with almost completely organic products. What happened? Urinary levels of six pesticide metabolites were measured before and after the change. A chemical called DAP fell by 89 percent after just one week of mostly organic food sourcing. Another chemical, called dimethylDAP, fell by 96 percent. The authors emphasized how quickly the body eliminates organophosphate pesticides when the diet is converted to organic produce and how this would be expected to enhance the health of the microbiome.

In a second study, a family of five was studied, including three children ages three to twelve.[4] They ate conventional foods for a week and then an organic diet for two weeks. During the organic phase they also changed household personal items to toxic-free brands. Urine was collected daily, and twelve different pesticides were assayed. The children in the family experienced a drop in pesticide excretion by over twelve times the baseline rate. Amazing. Overall, a ninefold drop was seen for the family as a whole. The changes occurred on the first day and were sustained for the two weeks.

Although studies on diet and autoimmune disease have not yet compared conventional to organic produce head to head, I would recommend considering the change in both food and personal products to limit toxins that may alter the microbiome and the immune response while providing all the advantages of plant-based nutrition.

CASE STUDY

Goodbye Lupus, Hello Plants

Brooke Goldner had been struggling with arthritis, horrific migraines, and a rash before she was diagnosed with systemic lupus erythematosus and advanced kidney failure at sixteen years old. The lupus was attacking her kidneys so aggressively that her doctors gave her six months before her kidneys would fail completely, leaving her on dialysis or dead. The only option they gave her to save her kidneys was to take chemotherapy to try to shut down her immune system. She endured the chemotherapy for two straight years in addition to steroids and other medications before she was considered in remission.

A week after her last chemotherapy treatment, she attended her first day of college and went on to graduate with honors and gain acceptance to medical schools. During that time, her lab tests still confirmed SLE, and she had some migraines, joint pains, and sensitivity to the sun, but was still considered stable.

During the stress of her third year of medical school, she had a mini-stroke due to the accelerated blood clots SLE can cause. She overcame the stroke and continued her training.

Around that time, she met her future husband, Thomas Tadlock, who was a celebrity trainer and fitness expert. At her request, he created a fitness program for her to look amazing at their wedding. He had to adjust the program he used for his clients because Brooke had been a long-time vegetarian and would not eat meat. She was, however, also a cheese addict, so she had to give up the dairy to get the rapid fat loss he was so famous for. Thus, accidentally, she ended up on a completely vegan nutrition plan, high in raw vegetables, omega-3s, and water, with no dairy, no meat, and no processed foods.

She quickly lost weight, going from a size 11 to a size 3 in only three and a half months. She also lost her joint pain, migraines, and fatigue. Four months later her lab tests for SLE were negative for the first time since she was diagnosed twelve years before that. Since that transformation in 2005, her laboratory studies have remained negative, an unheard-of full remission. Brooke went on to complete her training in psychiatry and neurology. Despite strongly worded advice to avoid pursuing pregnancy with SLE, she had two uneventful pregnancies and healthy children. When the lupus did not come back after pregnancy and childbirth, she and her husband realized the lupus was not coming back.

Both of them being scientists, they decided to investigate what could have caused this dramatic healing that was considered impossible, according to Western medicine. They realized that the only thing they had changed was Brooke's diet and spent the next two years reverse engineering everything she ate while she healed, as well as everything she had given up, and how her new diet could have impacted her cellular health and her immune function. They came to realize that they had accidentally created the most anti-inflammatory diet possible and began constructing a nutrition protocol that they would go on to successfully test on other people with autoimmune disease. Every person they treated had positive results, and many came off medications completely. In 2013, Dr. Brooke Goldner retired from her position as medical director of a nonprofit clinic to dedicate herself fully to educating doctors and patients about how to reverse chronic disease using supermarket foods.

Now, years later, she continues to eat a whole-food, plant-based diet of both cooked and raw foods with lots of green smoothies, soups, stews, and black bean burgers. She has a full online medical practice and also counsels patients with chronic disease.

In 2015, she wrote her bestselling book, *Goodbye Lupus*, documenting her amazing recovery. The book provides an easy-to-follow guide for how to use food to heal disease. Dr. Goldner has inspired many and plans to continue to tell her story and teach others about the power of plants to heal the body from even the most severe illnesses like SLE. ■

Thyroid Disease

The thyroid gland has a propensity to be involved in the autoimmune wars. Thyroid disease is very common and much of it is autoimmune. Autoimmune thyroid disease means antibody-mediated damage to the thyroid that can result in overactivity (hyperthyroidism) or underactivity (hypothyroidism) of the gland. An estimated 4 percent of men have some type of autoimmune thyroid disease, and it is much more common in women. As many as 5 million people in the United States alone may have this clinical problem. It is often found in families that have other autoimmune diseases.

The prevalence of the overactive thyroid gland associated with dietary pattern was examined in the Adventist Health Study.[5] Over

65,000 church members provided demographic, dietary, lifestyle, and medical history data by questionnaire. The prevalence of self-reported hyperthyroidism was 9 percent. Male gender and moderate or high income protected against hyperthyroidism, while obesity and cardiovascular disease were associated with increased risk. Vegan, lacto-ovo (dairy, eggs, and plants), and pesco (fish and plants) vegetarian diets were associated with lower risk compared with omnivorous diets, with vegan diets being the most protective and lowering the risk of hyperthyroidism by 50 percent. The authors concluded that eliminating all animal foods was associated with half the prevalence of hyperthyroidism compared with omnivorous diets. So what are you waiting for?

Another study from the Adventist Health Study examined hypothyroidism.[6] This is the condition where the thyroid gland produces too little thyroid hormone, and the metabolism slows. Diet was examined in over 65,000 participants. Vegan versus omnivorous diets tended to be associated with reduced risk of hypothyroidism by about 11 percent while a lacto-ovo diet was associated with increased risk of the condition by about the same amount. Following a vegan diet tended to be protective against hypothyroidism. Again, protect your thyroid, your heart, your brain, and your joints by following the Plant-Based Solution.

Plant Rant

We clearly need more medical studies about the Plant-Based Solution and autoimmune disorders. Moreover, the current therapies are often extremely expensive and are associated with side effects that can be very severe or even lethal. With a wealth of data that dairy and meat can provoke an inflammatory response, a plant-based therapy, like that followed by Dr. Brooke Goldner, is highly recommended. Those who advocate butter in coffee, bone broth, and full-fat dairy have simply no evidence that demonstrates a healing impact on autoimmune diseases. Heal your immune system and stop the war by following the Plant-Based Solution.

THE PLANT-BASED PLAN **Make Your Own Salad Dressing**

Homemade salad dressing is quick and easy to make and much healthier than most store-bought dressings. Feel free to get creative with this basic recipe. It makes about 1⅓ cups of dressing.

SALAD DRESSING

INGREDIENTS

½   cup freshly squeezed lemon juice

3   tablespoons balsamic vinegar

2   tablespoons mustard of choice

1   tablespoon maple syrup

½   teaspoon freshly ground pepper

OPTIONAL ADD-INS

Finely chopped shallots, minced herbs, and/or garlic

INSTRUCTIONS

1. In a container with a tight-fitting lid, combine the lemon juice, balsamic vinegar, mustard, maple syrup, and freshly ground pepper.

2. Shake well and store in the refrigerator. Remember to remove the dressing from the refrigerator 20 to 30 minutes before you want to use it.

10

Plant-Powered GI and Kidney Systems

am lumping gut and kidney health together because pee and poop just seem like a natural fit. More studies on disease reversal akin to those done on heart diseases and cancer are needed. Nonetheless, whenever you choose a WFPB meal for your heart, prostate, and brain, you will also be treating your kidneys and GI system to a healthy experience.

I discussed the microbiome in prior chapters and how the Plant-Based Solution favors bacterial colonies that promote insulin sensitivity. I also explained the causation between processed red meat and colorectal cancer. The production of TMAO by gut bacteria and the impact on cardiac and kidney health is familiar to you now. The champion status of vegans and bowel movement frequency was reviewed with the discussion on Parkinson's disease. This chapter will emphasize other important GI- and kidney-related topics.

CASE STUDY

Curing Ulcerative Colitis with the Plant-Based Solution

Like many college athletes, Kenny was focused on packing in foods rich in animal proteins—spicy buffalo wings, curly fries, raw eggs, and chocolate milk—to fill out and compete in football. Junk food was fine with him. It all fell apart a few years ago when he was rushed to the hospital with rectal bleeding and abdominal pain during his freshman college year. He required blood transfusions and was diagnosed with ulcerative colitis. He was treated with steroids. He experienced major weight loss from the inflammation in his colon. His dreams of a football career seemed crushed.

Kenny received little nutrition advice from his medical team, but other patients mentioned a WFPB diet as an option. Kenny would not give up on his dreams so he read everything he could on diet and GI health. He decided to adopt a vegan diet that was rich in fruit. Some days he would eat eighteen bananas a day. Other food staples were mangoes, dates, papayas, potatoes, and rice. Within a month he had gained ten pounds, felt fit, and was back on the team. Within a year, all lab tests and symptoms had normalized, and his doctors could not find any traces left of colitis. Furthermore, his weight returned to normal while he worked out, and he bulked up with plant-based muscle.

Now Kenny is ripped and feels great. He is often seen eating a plate-ful of baked potatoes with guacamole and steamed broccoli. Other days some beans and rice, vegetable bowls, and even Pad Thai without egg will fill him up. When we talked, he said, "I thought I would never be able to give up meat or dairy and that it would be a constant battle to not be tempted to eat a steak here and there, but in reality I don't miss it. I am more than happy with the food I am eating and have no intentions of going back. A vegan lifestyle has saved my life and healed all traces of the disease ulcerative colitis." ■

Study In-Depth: Animal-Based Foods and Gut Health

Inflammatory bowel disease (IBD), like the ulcerative colitis that Kenny suffered from, afflicts many people. Diet is rarely mentioned as either a potential cause or a potential treatment pathway. A large study in France sought to investigate if there might be a connection between meat-based diets and IBD.[1]

Among 67,581 participants followed for many years, seventy-seven developed new cases of IBD. High total protein intake, specifically animal protein, was associated with a significantly increased risk of IBD. In fact, there was three times higher risk for those who ate the most total protein and specifically animal protein. Among sources of animal protein, high consumption of meat or fish was associated with

IBD risk. High protein intake is also associated with an increased risk of incident IBD in French middle-aged women.

Science Corner: The Plant-Based Solution and Colon Health

The dramatic case of Kenny and his IBD is powerful but not unique. A thirty-six-year-old man who adopted a low-carb diet patterned after the Atkins diet began to lose weight but noticed bloody stools. A colonoscopy revealed diffuse inflammation limited to the rectum, and the man was diagnosed with ulcerative colitis. He was aware of data on plant-based diets and IBD and was provided a diet free of meat during his hospitalization. His bloody stools disappeared, and he achieved remission without medication for inflammatory bowel disease. This case indicates that an onset of ulcerative colitis can be an adverse event with a low-carbohydrate weight-loss diet.

Growing Healthy Guts with Plants

The Japanese medical community has adopted plant-based diets for IBD with more consistency than other health communities. A large study was performed using a semi-vegetarian diet for the prevention of Crohn's disease relapse.[2] In a single medical center over two years, sixteen adult patients with Crohn's in clinical remission consumed a semi-vegetarian diet after hospitalization. Remission was maintained in fifteen of the sixteen patients (94 percent) in the diet group versus two of six patients (33 percent) in the omnivorous group. Remission rate in the diet-compliant group was 100 percent after one year and 92 percent after two years. A blood test for inflammation was normal at the final visit in more than half of the patients in remission who were compliant with the diet. Overall, it appeared that the diet was highly effective in preventing relapse of IBD.

As discussed earlier, the World Health Organization announced in October 2015 that processed red meats can cause cancer. An additional few words on the topic are in order in view of a large analysis of diets and cancer.[3] The Adventist Health Study assessed the association between dietary patterns (non-vegetarian, lacto-, pesco-, vegan-, and semi-vegetarian) and the overall cancer incidence among 69,120 participants; 2,939 incident cancer cases were identified. A statistically significant association was found between a vegetarian diet and cancers of the gastrointestinal tract, with nearly a 25 percent reduction in the rates of these cancers in the vegetarians. Vegan diets showed statistically significant protection for overall cancer incidence of over 15 percent in men and women and by over 30 percent for female-specific cancers. On the whole, a vegan diet seems to confer lower risk for overall and female-specific cancer than other dietary patterns.

Diverticular disease, particularly diverticulitis, results in abdominal pain, fever, bowel dysfunction, and many emergency room visits requiring labs, CT scans, antibiotics, and occasionally surgery. While the medical community may be excellent at addressing the problem, what about the root cause? Fiber, which is present only in plant-based foods and not in any animal-based foods, is the key to great gut health and prevention of this problem. It is timely to mention the important contributions of Dennis Burkitt, MD, an English physician who spent many years practicing medicine in Africa. His experience in Uganda led him to make observations that were decades ahead of his time. There, he hardly ever saw anyone with the most common diseases in the United States and England, including coronary heart disease, adult-onset diabetes, varicose veins, obesity, diverticulitis, appendicitis, gallstones, dental cavities, hemorrhoids, hiatus hernias, and constipation. The Ugandan diet was simple and plant-based. He recalled removing only one gallbladder in twenty years in Africa.

In addition to discovering that one of the most common cancers in African children was due to an Epstein-Barr viral infection (known as Burkitt lymphoma), Dr. Burkitt's other major contribution was focusing on the role of dietary fiber to promote health. He wrote a bestselling book, *Don't Forget Fibre in Your Diet to Help Avoid Many of Our Commonest Diseases*, in 1979 that influenced the thinking of many health authorities and the food industry. He gets credit for placing plant-based fiber as a central pillar of disease prevention.

The EPIC-Oxford study in the United Kingdom examined over 47,000 men and women for dietary patterns and the development of diverticular disease.[4] Dietary fiber was estimated by food diaries. With a follow-up time of twelve years, there were 812 cases of diverticular disease including six deaths. Vegetarians had a 31 percent lower risk of diverticular disease compared with meat eaters. The probability of admission to a hospital or death from diverticular disease between the ages of fifty and seventy for meat eaters was 4.4 percent compared with 3 percent for vegetarians. Study participants with the highest intake of fiber (>25 grams daily) had a 41 percent lower risk compared with those in the lowest group (<14 grams daily). Overall, consuming a vegetarian diet and a high intake of dietary fiber were both associated with a lower risk of admission to a hospital or death from diverticular disease. Looks like Dr. Burkitt was right, whether in Uganda, the United Kingdom, or the United States.

Kidney Disease

It is time to turn to kidney disease and your health. As the kidneys go, so goes overall health. Kidney health is crucial for overall health, and when they weaken, all systems suffer. The spilling of protein in the urine is a sensitive early test for generalized kidney failure and specifically renal endothelial dysfunction. The simple MACR (microalbumin-to-creatinine ratio) test is what improved dramatically in Adam in just thirty days on a WFPB diet (see chapter 6).

An advantage of vegan diets on renal function has been formally studied, and the MACR measurement has been confirmed to be lower with a plant-based diet.[5] In fact, increased spilling of protein in the urine as an early sign of kidney damage has been directly associated with dietary animal fat and the consumption of meat.[6] In a sub-study of the Nurses' Health Study, 3,348 women had data at baseline and follow-up for MACR along with dietary histories. In women eating the highest amount of animal fat, the risk of developing urinary protein (called proteinuria) was almost twice as high as those eating lower amounts of animal fat.[7] In addition, in the nurses eating two or more servings of red meat per week, there was a 150 percent increase in developing proteinuria. To be kind to your kidneys, you may want to be kind to the animals too and choose plants.

In addition to the above factors for kidney disease, diabetes mellitus and hypertension are two potent forces that damage kidney health. The role of WFPB diets in those conditions has been discussed previously. By preventing diabetes and hypertension, the burden of advanced kidney disease would dramatically shrink.

Dietary recommendations to prevent and manage advanced kidney diseases are complex and require considerations of protein sources, phosphorus accumulation, calcium, and other factors. There is at least some basis to recommend a WFPB diet to patients already suffering from chronic kidney disease (CKD). In a small trial of such patients, a meat-based diet was compared to a grain- and soy- and plant-based diet in terms of phosphorus levels and hormone production affecting calcium metabolism.[8] Over a seven-day diet period, the plant-based patients had lower serum phosphorus levels. Their hormone levels also decreased in a favorable direction. Overall, the choice of plant-based protein had a significant effect on phosphorus homeostasis in patients with CKD. The better tolerance of the grain and soy diet suggested that dietary protein restrictions that are imposed in patients with CKD might be able to be revised, focusing on plant-based protein sources.

Ever have a kidney stone? Kidney stones cause the worst pain of a lifetime, in most people's opinion. Rather than treat them, why not prevent them with a WFPB diet? The EPIC-Oxford study examined the frequency of new kidney stones requiring hospital admission in over 51,000 participants.[9] Compared to those with a high intake of meat (>100 grams per day), the risk for vegetarians was nearly 40 percent lower. High intakes of fresh fruit and fiber from whole grains were also associated with a lower risk of kidney stone formation. That vegetarians may have a lower risk of developing kidney stones compared with those who eat a high-meat diet should motivate many who have felt the pain of a kidney stone to follow the Plant-Based Solution.

Plant Rant

There is nothing sexy or macho about picturing a caveman on dialysis. Kidney disease has weakened some of my patients, aged their arteries and body, and often shortens their lifespan and healthspan. The ideas that meat and animal fats are needed for muscle development and brain health, that we need more and more animal protein particularly from grilled chicken, and that plant-based proteins are somehow inadequate are all doing great harm to many. An elephant eats plants. A gorilla eats predominantly plants. A horse pulls six people and eats hay and oats. Muscle develops just fine with the amino acids that make up the proteins in plant-based foods because they are the same amino acids as in animal muscle. Lysine is lysine no matter where it comes from. Just check out a vegan body builder website if you have any doubt about the potential to feed a rough and tough muscular man or woman on fruits, vegetables, legumes, nuts, and seeds alone.

THE PLANT-BASED PLAN Try a Probiotic Food to Support Your Microbiome

The availability of probiotic foods has exploded in recent years. Natural food stores offer a variety of options, and some are easy to make at home too. See if you can find one or more that you like to include in your daily diet:

- Fermented vegetables, like sauerkraut and kimchi

- Sour pickles (check the label to confirm they contain probiotics)

- Kombucha, a fermented tea beverage

- Kvass, a fermented vegetable and/or fruit beverage

- Nondairy yogurts (made from soy, coconut, or almond milk)

- Water kefir, a fermented beverage made from flavored water, juice, or coconut water

- Miso (use as an ingredient in recipes for dressings, sauces, soups, and more)

11

Fifty Shades of Green
with Plants and Sex

You do not need to keep this book wrapped in a brown paper cover, but let's have some real conversation here. I hope this is the section of the book most highlighted and with the most page corners turned over. I hate to burst your bubble so early in the chapter, but we have more bravado and testimonials of enhanced sexual prowess on plant-based diets than we have peer-reviewed scientific reports. The most famous may be the scene in the movie *Forks Over Knives*, where reference is made to the ability to "raise the flag" again on a plant-based diet. There is also an accompanying video on the topic of plants and sexual power that gained considerable public attention.[1] There is every reason to believe that the Plant-Based Solution is the most reliable path to male and female potency for as long as possible, and the science as it exists supports that notion.

For the estimated 30 million men in the United States with erectile dysfunction (ED), both their romantic lives and their heart health can suffer. In fact, research shows that ED can be an early warning sign of heart disease. Not only are both endothelial (blood vessel) dysfunction and erectile dysfunction "ED," but they are related, as you will see. When there is endothelial dysfunction, there is usually at least some erectile dysfunction. Around 300 years ago, Ben Franklin wrote that an ounce of prevention is worth a pound of cure. Similarly, I often tell my male patients "to be older and hard, exercise and eat no lard!"

CASE STUDY
Stiff Evidence for a Plant-Based Diet

Stan's heart scare was a blessing in disguise. His text to me that he was having a strange feeling in his chest while exerting himself at the gym alarmed me. When a sixty-year-old man says those words, the diagnosis of a badly clogged heart artery is over 90 percent likely. It had been only a few weeks of having the feeling of two to three minutes of fullness in the chest, which quickly resolved with rest, something called classic angina. Stan came to my office the same day, and his EKG was abnormal. I arranged an urgent cardiac catheterization, and two of his major heart arteries were 95 percent clogged. The third had disease, but it was moderate. He received two stents in the hospital and went home uneventfully.

On his first follow-up visit, he was doing fine; all of his symptoms had resolved. He was a very educated man and came with a list of questions based on his careful Internet research. He was in the health-care field himself but admitted to not placing his health as a priority. Exercise had been rare, his weight had steadily crept up over a quarter century of practice as a health-care consultant, and his sleep was interrupted by loud snoring, which he ignored. He also indicated that he had bothersome erectile dysfunction, which he attributed to age and stress.

His decision to adopt the Plant-Based Solution was immediate, and he was struck by a presentation by Dr. Caldwell Esselstyn he watched on YouTube while still in the hospital recovering from his stents. He also read several other books and visited many health websites. He began a twenty-one-day immersion into plant-based eating without added oils and found it satisfying. He entered a Pritikin Intensive Cardiac Rehabilitation program locally where he took plant-based nutrition, cooking, and exercise classes. He said goodbye to his old diet and was 100 percent on board with the only heart disease reversal diet ever proven to work, a plant-based, no-added-oil program.

At his three-month visit, he was beaming with pride as the scale showed a fourteen-pound weight loss, and he felt great. His fasting blood sugars no longer ran 120 and were in the low 80s, which is normal. He was about to finish cardiac rehabilitation and was looking forward to working out at the local gym with renewed confidence and stamina. Stan was most excited, however, by his restored ability to obtain and maintain an erection without the blue pills. He said it was "a zillion" times better. He told me that he had told his buddies, many of whom had erectile dysfunction, that "Spanish fly was overrated—all you have to do is eat like a gorilla." ■

The Sexiest Foods Are Plant-Based

An estimated 300 million men worldwide will soon suffer from erectile dysfunction,[2] and most of those men will also be at risk for heart disease and stroke. Fruit may be part of the solution.

Researchers from Harvard Medical School performed the first observational study of dietary habits and sexual function over a ten-year period. The study concentrated on flavonoid intake from plant-based foods disclosed on food-frequency questionnaires collected every four years. Over 25,000 participants rated their erectile function in 2000 and again in 2004 and 2008.[3]

During ten years of follow-up, 36 percent of the men reported ED. After analyzing other factors like smoking and diabetes (classic cardiovascular disease risk factors), several classes of dietary flavonoids—flavones, anthocyanins, and flavanones—were associated with reduced ED. A higher intake of flavanones, anthocyanins, and flavones was significantly associated with a reduction in risk of ED in men younger than seventy years old, but not older men. A higher total intake of fruit, a major source of anthocyanins and flavanones, was associated with a 14 percent reduction in risk of ED. It is now widely appreciated that erectile dysfunction is often an early barometer of poor vascular function and offers a critical opportunity to intervene and prevent cardiovascular disease, heart attack, and even death.

I would advise you to not wait until you're dealing with ED to take charge of your health. Avoidance of ED can be added to numerous other benefits of adopting the Plant-Based Solution.

Prevent ED with Flavonoid-Rich Foods

Add fruit to keep the blue pill away. Data suggest that a higher habitual intake of specific flavonoid-rich foods is associated with reduced ED incidence. Preserve your sexual responsiveness by including these foods in your meals: apples, blueberries, citrus, pears, red wine, and strawberries.

Science Corner: The Hard Truth about Sexy Plants

Katherine Esposito, MD, of Naples, Italy, has done a series of studies on the Mediterranean diet and erectile dysfunction. While the MED diet often advises fish over red meat and is not a fully plant-based pattern, it is a very plant-strong model to study, and there are many people who follow a "vegiterranean" version. In one study, the effect of a Mediterranean-style diet on ED in men was examined.[4] The sixty-five men in the study had ED and also the metabolic syndrome, which includes abdominal obesity, high cholesterol or triglycerides, high blood pressure, and an elevated blood sugar that together predict increased cardiac risk. Thirty-five of them were assigned to the Mediterranean-style diet and thirty to the control diet. After two years, men on the Mediterranean diet consumed more fruits, vegetables, nuts, whole grains, and olive oil as compared with men on the control diet. Inflammatory blood markers like the C-reactive protein improved in the MED diet group but were unchanged in the control group. There were thirteen men in the MED diet group and two in the control group that reported improved ED measures. The study suggested that a Mediterranean-style diet rich in whole grains, fruits, vegetables, legumes, walnuts, and olive oil might be effective in reducing the prevalence of ED in men with the metabolic syndrome.

The Endothelium and ED

How are flavonols and other plant-based foods able to boost the sexual response? Recall from chapter 2 that inside every blood vessel is a single-cell lining called the endothelium, and this layer of cells makes that miraculous chemical called nitric oxide. The production of NO leads to the creation of a compound called cyclic GMP. To get blood rushing and swelling to the sexual parts involved, lots of NO is needed. In fact, the erectile dysfunction drugs that you see advertised on TV also work by increasing cyclic GMP levels.

How is nitric oxide generated in these key blood vessels? The amino acids L-arginine and L-citrulline cycle back and forth and create it. This system is particularly active before the age of forty. If you want to boost levels of NO, eat healthy foods high in L-arginine, such as pine nuts, peanuts, walnuts, almonds, pistachios, and Brazil nuts. Grains, including oats and wheat germ, also have significant amounts of L-arginine.

I mentioned the amino acid citrulline above and how it can help arteries support romance and passion. Where do you find it? Watermelon has the highest concentration of citrulline (particularly the white rind) in nature, followed by onions and garlic. You might want to stick to watermelon, however, before going on a date! Yellow watermelon has even more citrulline than red melon. Remember that there is a second way to generate NO and its blood flow–enhancing effects. Chemicals called dietary nitrates found in many foods (like greens and beets) are converted in our saliva to nitrites, absorbed, and then converted to NO. Antiseptic mouthwashes prevent this healthy conversion and should be avoided if you want the benefit of plant-based dietary NO boosters.

Arugula, rhubarb, kale, Swiss chard, spinach, bok choy, and beets are at the top of the list of plant-based sources of dietary nitrates. If you also try to add grapes, pomegranates, apples, and green teas to your diet, you have a dynamite erotic potion.

Over 400 years ago, English physician Thomas Sydenham said, "A man is as old as his arteries." Four centuries later, we know just how right he was and that it is not only men who benefit. Women also need blood flow for romance, and the same systems work in the female body, although women are studied less often in research protocols.

Plant Rant

Some men like to brag about their sexual prowess, whether in the gym or the bedroom. It seems that the Paleo movement has done a better job of presenting shirtless and confident men as representatives of a diet that is often heavily meat-based and deflating to arteries and the sexual response. In reality, the sexiest man is the one holding a baby lamb or chicken saved from slaughter and not eating it. And that man probably has preserved sexual responsiveness due to the concentration of plant-based nutrients that promote vascular health, NO production, and sexual competency. While more research is needed, the best blue pill is a blueberry. The best aphrodisiac is a person in tune with kindness to animals, the confidence knowing the environment is suffering as little as possible by wise plant-based food choices made, and sexually powered with plant-fueled genitals.

THE PLANT-BASED PLAN   Try a Meal-Kit Delivery Service or Take a Cooking Class

You've probably noticed the trend in meal-kit delivery services—those that deliver a box of premeasured, and often precut, ingredients with recipes to your home. Purple Carrot (purplecarrot.com) is one such service that offers vegan options. Don't want to cook at all? Sakara (sakara.com) delivers fully prepared vegan meals to your door.

When new patients begin the Plant-Based Solution, one of the first things I do is suggest a cooking class. Culinary Rx (plantricianrouxbe.com) offers a plant-based online cooking course for $99.

12

The Garden of Youth

Lifespan is determined by about 10 percent genetic makeup and 90 percent lifestyle. The best lifestyle for the goals of enjoying both a long lifespan and a long healthspan appears to be following the Plant-Based Solution. It is sound advice that if you want something in life, find people who've accomplished that goal and learn from them, like adventurer and bestselling author Dan Buettner.

Buettner's 2005 cover story for *National Geographic*, "The Secrets of Living Longer," was a finalist for a National Magazine Award. For that story, Buettner proposed finding communities where people lived to be over 100 with regularity. He highlighted the areas verified as zones of longevity (dubbed "Blue Zones" for the blue marker he used on a world map to confirm a longevity zone), and he found five areas: (1) Okinawa, Japan; (2) Loma Linda, California; (3) Sardinia, Italy; (4) Nicoya, Costa Rica; and (5) Ikaria, Greece. He found common patterns among these Blue Zones even though they were very far from one another. These included an absence of smoking, daily physical activity centered on walking, a plant-heavy diet with very small amounts of animal foods, strong family connections, and strong social connections. For example, in Loma Linda, California, home of the Seventh-day Adventist Church, vegetarianism is a celebrated lifestyle, and eating nuts is common. In Okinawa, Japan, it is taught that you should eat until you are 80 percent full, and the average daily food intake there is hundreds of calories less than in other parts of Japan. In Sardinia they have the ultra-powerful Cannonau wine, in Ikaria boiled coffee, and in Costa Rica unlimited supplies of fresh tropical fruit. The idea that a diet based on plants, along with other lifestyle measures, may prolong life has quite a bit of scientific support.

The Connection Between Lifestyle and Aging

One way to estimate the biological age of a person is to examine the tips of the person's chromosomes. The caps at the end of DNA molecules are called telomeres (often compared to the tips of shoelaces), and they protect the genetic DNA material from damage. The length of the telomere determines the number of times a cell can divide before failing and therefore is related to longevity.

Not only did Dr. Dean Ornish do landmark research on heart disease reversal and prostate cancer, he also tackled longevity. Dr. Ornish joined forces with 2009 Nobel Prize winner Elizabeth Blackburn, PhD, to work with him on aging. The team, led by Blackburn, discovered an enzyme called telomerase that maintains the telomeres as long as possible. Ornish and Blackburn were curious about whether the activity of telomerase was influenced by lifestyle. They wondered if a healthy lifestyle made the telomeres longer, slowing aging or even reversing it.

Ornish and Blackburn studied thirty-five men with low-risk prostate cancer who were randomized to the lifestyle program or a control group for five years. The ten men in the treatment group ate a diet of plants, did not smoke, walked daily for fitness, managed stress with yoga and meditation, and had social support and love from support groups. When they measured the activity of telomerase, they found it increased in activity in the lifestyle group after only three months. After five years, there was a significant 10 percent increase in telomere length in the lifestyle group, whereas the length got shorter in the control group.[1] This was the first controlled study showing that any intervention may lengthen telomeres, thereby beginning to reverse aging at a cellular level. The study's finding was hailed as a breakthrough on aging and lifestyle, and the implications for extending life by healthy habits are huge. As telomere length would be expected to shorten with time, the potential to reverse this process, and possibly reversing aging, was enthusiastically embraced. The best antiaging program begins with wise use of your fork and spoon.

CASE STUDY

Ellsworth Wareham, MD, Heart Surgeon

Ellsworth Wareham, MD, has inspired many people, including neurosurgeon and reporter Sanjay Gupta of CNN who interviewed him as he approached his one hundredth birthday. Now 102, Dr. Wareham attributes his longevity to his vegan diet. He powers his day with vegetables from his garden, does his own yardwork, and is up and down stairs in his home in Loma Linda, California (the seat of the Seventh-day Adventist Church).

A World War II navy veteran who won many awards, he was one of the earliest physicians trained as a cardiac surgeon in the United States. He adopted a vegan diet over forty years ago after examining thousands of clogged arteries directly and studying the causes. He concluded that animal products raise cholesterol, and he decided to get his down. He says that if blood cholesterol is kept under 150, the chances of getting a heart attack are very low. His cholesterol is 117. Think of Dr. Wareham if you happened to read that you need a lot of cholesterol for proper brain function. He eats none with his plant-based diet, and despite his low cholesterol, he is sharp as can be.

Dr. Wareham retired from cardiac surgery at age seventy-four but taught residents and assisted them for another twenty-one years. His garden is his passion, and he wakes up at 5:00 a.m. after eight hours of sleep, exercises, spends time with his family, and tends to his plants. He mows his own lawn. A typical breakfast is whole-wheat cereal and almond milk. He does not need a cane or walker and has a goal of climbing twenty flights of stairs a week. He is a remarkable example of plant-powered aging. ■

How Food Affects Genes

What if your family history of heart disease or cancer is bad? Aren't our genes our destiny when it comes to aging and chronic diseases? Or do we have control over the majority of health issues based on our lifestyle habits? In 2003, the entire human genome was sequenced for the first time. When the number of genes in human cells were counted and compared to other organisms, our genome was considerably smaller than that of many other species. For example, humans have about 25,000 genes in each cell, while the tiny water flea has over 30,000 genes! Scientists had previously assumed that our advanced abilities and organ structure would be associated with many more genes than that.

While we don't have as many genes as expected, scientists have discovered that humans have very complex ways to control the modest number of genes we have. This is an exciting new field called epigenetics. Epigenetics explains how changes in gene activity can occur without changing our actual DNA. One way that we can influence genes without changing their basic structure is through the foods we eat. This is often called nutrigenomics. I teach patients that our genes load the gun, but our lifestyle pulls the trigger. Our fork is so powerful that it not only transports food to our mouth, but it also can be used to turn genetic activity on and off.

To date, the most impressive studies on nutrigenomics have been performed with the Ornish Lifestyle Medicine Program, as you have read. Here is a brief summary of two of the studies showing the ability to control our gene activity, and perhaps longevity, with a plant-based lifestyle.

A PLANT-BASED DIET CAN TURN OFF PROSTATE CANCER GENES

A low-fat WFPB diet along with stress management, walking, and social support in thirty-one men with low-grade prostate cancer was found after only three months to increase the activity of 48 genes involved in cancer control while decreasing the activity of 453 genes (ones that controlled for tumor growth and protein production).[2] These epigenetic changes from the lifestyle plan were associated with shrinking the size of the prostate cancers.

A PLANT-BASED DIET IMPROVES GENES, CONTROLLING INFLAMMATION, WEIGHT, AND VASCULAR HEALTH

In a study conducted in Pennsylvania, sixty-three individuals with heart disease who followed the Ornish program were compared to a group of sixty-three people who did not follow any particular program.[3] The group following the Ornish lifestyle program lost weight and their blood pressure fell by about 10 percent, unlike the control group. What was amazing was that after just three months on the program, twenty-six genes were exhibiting different activity in the lifestyle group. After a year, 143 genes were measured to have different activity. The genes that promoted inflammation and blood-vessel injury were significantly reduced in activity. The control group showed no improvements. The study showed that you can control the activity of your genes through lifestyle and have at least partial control of aging, cancer, and blood-vessel damage.

The power of epigenetics is enormous. In fact, lifestyle medicine should always be offered before or along with conventional therapies. Food is information and can be viewed as a remote control to our genes, turning them on and off by a variety of modifications. Our fork and spoon are the most powerful surgical instruments there are. Load up your plate with a pile of rainbow-colored, whole-food plants and enjoy the odds of a life free of illness and medications. You might just find that smoother skin and a bounce in your step are just a forkful away.

Hot Question: Where Do You Get Your Protein?

This is the number-one question a vegan is asked most frequently. Not how do you feel, why do you look so good, where is your energy from, how does it feel to be kind to animals, or are you proud of sustaining the earth? It is always about protein. So, here are a few words on a topic that is a myth and probably stems from the meat and dairy industries' fear of their livelihoods being transferred to plant-based suppliers of foods.

There are so many sources of plant-based proteins that only an extremely restricted diet could ever pose a problem. Even athletes who follow a form of diet that is mainly fruit and low in protein thrive in competition and have incredible endurance. For example, 100 percent whole grains and legumes are good plant-based protein sources. Greens like kale and collard greens are rich in protein. Foods like tempeh and organic tofu are worth trying and are easily available. Seitan, aka wheat gluten, contains just as much protein as beefsteak.

If you like to measure things, you can calculate how much protein you might need on average. It is recommended that you eat about 0.75 to 1.0 gram of protein per kilogram of body weight daily, so if you weigh 220 pounds, or 100 kilograms, that is about 80 to 100 grams of protein. As an example, to eat about 80 grams of plant-based protein in a day, you would need to eat about 1 kg, or 4 bowls, of beans, lentils, or chickpeas in soups, salads, hummus, and casseroles.

A diet comprising a variety of plant protein sources will include all the essential amino acids you need. There are some plant-based foods that do contain all the essential amino acids, such as soy, buckwheat, quinoa, and amaranth. You do not need to eat complete proteins at each meal. Your body can store and combine the essential amino acids.

Plant-based sources of protein:

- Legumes: peas; beans (adzuki beans, black-eyed peas, chickpeas including chickpea flour, kidney beans); lentils; soy foods (tofu, tempeh, soy milk)

- Nuts: cashews, almonds, peanuts, pistachios

- Seeds: pumpkin, sunflower, sesame, chia

- Grains: 100 percent whole-wheat, oats, buckwheat, millet, quinoa, amaranth, pasta, bread

Smoother Skin: Bone Broth or Bean Broth?

A current food fad crossing the world is the idea that ingesting the collagen, marrow, and broth of cooked animal bones fulfills our ancestral needs and is a fast track to GI health, weight loss, and glowing skin. If I had a dollar for every time bone broth has been called a miracle on the Internet . . .

A recent survey of the medical literature searching for health benefits from bone broth found an important article. Animals and humans often store toxic lead within bone minerals. In 2013, scientists measured the levels of lead in broth made from the bones of organic chickens.[4] The broth was found to have markedly high lead concentrations compared to water (cooked in the same cookware). Beware the broth. Do any commercially available bone broths or collagen powders test for lead levels? Furthermore, humans cannot absorb collagen. If there is any nutrition derived from the broth, it is because enzymes break the protein down to amino acids, just like plant protein sources, and reformat them in individual cells to make proteins dictated by the activity of our DNA.

If you want a natural approach to healthy skin, it is important to learn that the human body requires vitamin C and the amino acid lysine to form collagen for healthy skin, arteries, and organs. Humans are unable to make both vitamin C and lysine and are completely dependent on dietary sources.

Linus Pauling, MD, a two-time Nobel Prize laureate and biochemist who lived into his nineties, theorized that both coronary artery disease and overall aging were due to a combination of a deficiency of vitamin C and lysine resulting in weakened arterial walls, skin structure, and organ health.[5] Why not increase food-based sources of vitamin C in your diet (citrus, other fruits, vegetables) and lysine (legumes and organic soy products) from whole-food sources for the health of your heart and the glow of your skin? I would recommend you bypass the bone broth.

Plant Rant

The popularity of the Paleo diet movement and the overlapping low-carb, high-fat diet movement is puzzling. There are no studies demonstrating favorable effects on our genome with these diets like there are with plant-based lifestyle programs. And there are no studies that demonstrate reversal of heart disease or the genetic activity that favors healthy arteries. With the abundance of data for WFPB diets, particularly when low in added fats, there is only one science-based choice. Eat a plant-based diet for the most antiaging benefits. (In a spirit of fairness, there is data that there may be favorable nutrigenomic responses to a Mediterranean diet rich in fruits, vegetables, legumes, and whole grains while being low in processed foods and red meat).[6]

THE PLANT-BASED PLAN Become an Expert Main-Dish-Salad Maker

A big salad is the perfect lunch (or dinner and even breakfast). It should be quick to prepare, and you can make unlimited variations. There is more to a main-dish salad than greens and raw veggies.

You can start with a base of greens if you wish, but it's not required. Mix it up. Try shredded kale, arugula, spinach, or even thinly sliced cabbage. You can add leftover roasted vegetables. Baked tofu, seeds, and nuts are good options too. A scoop of hummus on top might sound unusual, but it goes great with a lemon-based dressing. Dried or fresh fruit—chopped apples, sliced strawberries, blueberries—is also terrific on salads. This is the perfect time to use your precooked beans, rice, and quinoa—use these items as a base with or instead of greens, or spoon them on top of greens. Don't forget your premade dressing (store-bought is fine too!).

13

Plants, the Plight of Animals, and World Religions

grew up in Detroit when two bottles of milk were delivered in the milk chute by the milk truck (yes, I am old enough to remember). Elsie the Cow was a symbol on bottles of a smiling cow, full udder brimming with fresh white milk that ended up on my kitchen table as a child. It all seemed so innocent, and I felt a bond with Elsie. I never pondered the life that Elsie had or the fact that my cold glass of milk may have been at the expense of her pain and that of her calves. It was a different age when transparency was not paramount.

The growth of the population and a drive to adopt the production-line model of automotive factories to animal farming has led to the shrinking of old-fashioned family farms and the rise of large and concentrated farming facilities. This practice has been termed "factory farming." (If you could do it for a Model T, why not a T-bone?) According to Last Chance for Animals, "factory farming is an industrial process in which animals and the products they generate are mass-produced. The animals are generally not seen as individual, sentient beings with unique physical and psychological needs but as eggs, milk, meat, leather, and other products to drive profits." Because the animals are seen as mere commodities, they are bred, fed, confined, and drugged to lay more eggs, birth more offspring, and die with more meat on their bones. The horrors caught on videos are gruesome. "Factory farms cut costs by feeding animals the remains of other animals, keeping them in extremely small and soiled enclosures and without adequate bedding. Animals that live in such a manner and are denied normal social interactions experience boredom and stress so great that it leads to unnatural aggression. To curb this aggression and to conceal the disease that results from such horrendous living conditions and stimulate aberrant growth, farmers routinely administer drugs to animals, which in turn reach meat-eating consumers. The consequences of this agribusiness amount to institutionalized animal cruelty, environmental destruction and resource depletion, and health dangers."[1]

The US Environmental Protection Agency describes large factory farms as concentrated animal feeding operations, or CAFOs.[2] There are over a quarter of a million animal feeding operations in the United States alone with over 15,000 of them large enough to be defined as a CAFO. The largest house, for example, has over 1,000 head of cattle. Livestock production has become increasingly dominated by CAFOs in the United States and other parts of the world. Most of the poultry consumed by humans began to be raised in CAFOs in the 1950s, and most cattle and pork CAFOs originated in the 1970s and 80s. CAFOs now dominate livestock and poultry production in the United States, and the scope of their market share is steadily increasing. For example, in 1966, it took 1 million farms to house 57 million pigs; by the year 2001, it only took 80,000 farms to house the same number of pigs.

Due to factors like the efficiency of CAFOs, the growth of the world population, the spread of fast-food restaurants worldwide, and the mixed messages from both social media and medical outlets that more meat may be healthier, the growth of animal production has been meteoric. Annually over 10 billion farm animals are produced and killed yearly with over 95 percent of them in a CAFO setting.

Are there ethical farmers? Those who love their animals until the day they are slaughtered? For sure there are, and they deserve recognition for opposing the more than 95 percent of factory-farmed foods that have a legacy of cruelty, disease, and worker injury. While some of the practices common to many factory farms today are unsettling, a consideration of their role in food production is necessary in understanding the full implications of choosing the Plant-Based Solution. A look at a few of the most common animals used for food production and how they fare in CAFOs is instructive, even if upsetting.

Beef Cattle

Cattle are frightened and confused when humans come to round them up and pack them onto trucks, and injuries often result. During transport, they are frightened, exposed to severe weather conditions, and deprived of food, water, and veterinary care. Cattle are then burned with a hot iron brand without anesthetic so that it is clear who "owns" them. Finally, they are castrated and dehorned without anesthetic.

Approximately 250 cows are killed every hour at the typical beef slaughterhouse. The animals are often treated rather cruelly. Although cattle are supposed to be rendered unconscious before being killed, workers frequently do not successfully "stun" the animals. As a result, conscious, struggling cows are hung upside down. Their throats are then cut.

Dairy Cows

Dairy cows live in crowded pens or barns with concrete floors. Milking machines often cut them and cause other injuries. Some machines give them electrical shocks, which cause extreme pain and even death. Dairy cows are forced to produce ten times more milk than they would produce in nature. As a result, they experience numerous health problems.

Veal Calves

Veal calves live in small wooden crates; some are chained. They cannot turn around or even stretch their legs. The floors of their stalls are slatted, causing them severe joint and leg pain. Since their mother's milk is taken for human consumption, they are fed a milk substitute deficient in iron and fiber. In other words, they are deliberately kept anemic, and their muscles are atrophied so that their flesh will be pale and tender. Craving iron, they lick the metallic parts of their stalls, even those covered in urine. Water is often withheld from them.

Pigs

Female pigs are kept pregnant continually. After being impregnated, sows are placed in eighteen- to twenty-inch-wide pens. There is barely enough room for them to stand up and lie down. Because straw is considered too expensive, they are not given bedding but instead forced to lie on hard floors, which, in part, cause crippling leg disorders. Sometimes they are tied to the floor by a chain or strap. The piglets are then taken away to be fattened up. By that time, approximately 15 percent of the newborns will have died. The sow is then reimpregnated, sometimes by being strapped to a table.

Broiler Chickens

Farmers get more money for chickens with enlarged thighs and breasts. As a result, they breed the animals to be so heavy that their bones cannot support their weight. The chickens have difficulty standing, and their legs often break. Like other factory-farmed animals, broiler chickens are raised in such overcrowded enclosures that they become aggressive. To stop them from fighting with one another, their beaks and toes are cut off without anesthetic. Some are injected with saltwater to pump up their flesh for sale, simultaneously driving the salt load in some chickens to dangerous levels.

Layer Chickens

Layer chickens lay 90 to 95 percent of all eggs sold in the United States. Newborn chicks are placed on a conveyor belt where a worker picks each one up to see if it is male or female. Newborn males are placed in trash bags and suffocated, decapitated, gassed, crushed, or ground up alive. Newborn females are placed back on the belt. The next worker then picks up the female chick, holds her up to a machine's hot iron that cuts off her beak, and then places her back on the belt. The beaks of these birds are removed because five to eight of them are crammed into fourteen-square-inch cages, cages so small that the birds cannot even spread their wings. Such close confinement, which averts their natural social order, causes aggression among the birds.

Turkeys

Turkeys are given less than three square feet of cage space. The ends of their beaks are cut off, and their toes are clipped, both without anesthesia. They are bred to be so heavy that their bones cannot support their weight. Moreover, they are so heavy that they cannot reproduce naturally. Consequently, they must be artificially inseminated.

Turkeys are loaded onto a conveyor belt. Some fall onto the ground instead of landing on the belt. Because workers are in such a rush, they rarely pick up those that have fallen. As a result, some birds die after being crushed by machinery operated near the unloading area. Others succumb to starvation and exposure. Inside the slaughterhouse, the turkeys are hung by their feet from metal shackles on a conveyor belt. Their heads are dunked in the stunning tank, an electrical bath of water.

Reprinted with permission from Last Chance for Animals, lcanimal.org.

CASE STUDY
Animal Rights Liberation Activist Gary Yourofsky

A few years ago, I sat down to dinner with a friend and was introduced to a man named Gary, who lived less than five minutes from where I was born. It took me about fifteen minutes to realize that he was Gary Yourofsky, the internationally celebrated animal activist with a YouTube video called "The Best Speech You Will Ever Hear," in which he compares our current treatment of animals to genocide. The talk was recorded at Georgia Tech in 2010 and has been viewed by millions of people.[3]

Gary had his life changed in his early twenties when his stepdad took him backstage at a local circus. He saw the animals chained and caged, and he reacted strongly to their cruel treatment. At the time, he ate anything anywhere. He began researching the production of his food and clothes. He realized that an "animal holocaust" was being tolerated unnecessarily, as plant-based diets provided all the nutrition humans need, and faux leathers were available. He decided to become an activist and has since been arrested thirteen times in his crusade to help animals. Most famously, he set 1,500 minks free from a farm in Ontario and was arrested and denied bail for ten days by a judge who had just granted bail in only one day to a sex offender. He ultimately served seventy-seven days in jail before being extradited. Today, Gary is banned from five countries, including Canada and the United Kingdom.

He has since been speaking to school groups and has given over 2,500 presentations to more than 60,000 people in more than thirty states, usually at high school and college campuses.

After Gary's 2010 YouTube video went viral, several animal rights activists translated it into Hebrew and posted it on Israeli websites. Plant-based groups and eateries are popular in Israel, and a buzz quickly developed. A website was created to popularize the YouTube video, and several vegetarian food manufacturers printed the link on their product labels. Gary was invited to speak in Israel and has since achieved cult status, with people recognizing and mobbing him on Israeli streets. Recent data indicates that over 15 percent of the Israeli nation is vegetarian (among the highest in the world). After Gary conducted a speaking tour of Israel in late 2013, dairy and meat sales fell by about 5 percent. Domino's Pizza in Israel announced they will start serving vegan pizzas. The largest state-owned dairy has a completely dairy-free line of products.[4] ∎

Science Corner: Ethical Veganism and Canadian Law

Raise your hand right now if you are or plan to be a health-based vegan? Keep your hand up. An ethical-based vegan? An environmental-based vegan? Everyone should have their hand up unless you are dating a vegan and just in it for romance and a romp! Actually, you do not need to declare your main goal of following the Plant-Based Solution, and you likely will find that all three reasons (health, ethics, and the environment) are strong arguments for never eating animal-based foods again. However, research has pointed out the importance of having a basis in ethical veganism to maintain this voluntary lifestyle long term. For instance, if you think of a hamburger as Elsie the Cow's ground-up thigh muscle after Elsie's life of misery with repeated insemination, infections, and confinement for milk production, you are far less likely to eat that hamburger than if you are motivated solely by achieving your optimal weight and cholesterol.

One interesting study researched the impact of whether 246 vegans were motivated primarily by ethical or health concerns and how that orientation influenced their journey toward the Plant-Based Solution.[5] The hypothesis was that compared to those following the diet for ethical reasons, those doing so for health reasons would consume foods with higher nutritional value and engage in other healthier lifestyle behaviors. Indeed, those citing health reasons reported eating more fruit and fewer sweets than did those citing ethical reasons. Other findings were that individuals endorsing primarily ethical reasons reported being on the diet longer and had a higher consumption of soy, foods rich in vitamin D, high-polyphenol beverages, and vitamin supplements (like D and B12) than did those endorsing health reasons. There's evidence to support the claim that people who become vegetarian or vegan for ethical reasons stick with it longer. Ethical vegans also frequently transition from vegetarian to vegan sooner than health-focused vegans.

It may strike you as odd, but advocating for the welfare of animals—even if you have not emptied out animal factories like Gary Yourofsky—has been challenging. The powerful meat and dairy industries often have legislation protecting them from those who try to make videos that expose the cruelty within their factory farms. The good news is that ethical beliefs are now protected under Ontario's human rights law as a form of "creed." Ontario's Human Rights Code protects people from discrimination based on their creed.[6]

The Ontario Human Rights Commission issued a much-awaited updated policy that defined creed as "non-religious belief systems that, like religion, substantially influence a person's identity, worldview and way of life."[7] This would include a belief system that seeks to avoid causing harm to animals, like ethical veganism. The policy recommends that a person in a hospital facility who has a creed-based need for vegetarian food be provided with appropriate food by the facility. Other protections included are: (1) Universities and schools have an obligation to accommodate students who refuse to perform animal dissections because of their creed; (2) employees do not have to wear animal-based components of a uniform, like leather or fur, based on their creed; and (3) an employer cannot exclude a vegetarian or vegan employee by, for example, holding regular company events at a steakhouse.[8]

Veganism and World Religions

Lessons of mercy to animals and respect for the planet found in many of the world religions are just one of the many paths that may lead you to choose a plant-based diet.

Judaism: In an early chapter of Genesis, it is written: "I give you every seed-bearing plant that is upon the earth, and every tree that has seed-bearing fruit; they shall be yours for food." The Book of Daniel is also viewed as a bedrock of religious support for vegetarianism. When the prophet Daniel and three fellow slaves were in captivity, they were offered the king's rich diet but refused and asked for only "vegetables to eat and water to drink." This verse has led to both a ten-day cleansing program and the highly successful lifestyle change program at the Saddleback Church in Southern California.[9]

Jewish dietary law stresses avoidance of cruelty to animals, whether in the production of food or as beasts of burden. The Jewish dietary laws of kosher and their Talmudic guidelines strive to create a more compassionate humanity. *Tza'ar ba'alei chayim* (the suffering of living creatures) is a Talmudic law that prevents unnecessary cruelty to all animals, including pets and livestock, and imposes specific obligations for those caring for animals. The ethical treatment of animals is a core Jewish value. In general, Judaism permits the eating of meat, provided the animal is a species permitted by the Torah and is ritually slaughtered. At the same time, the Torah stresses compassion for animals, such as not causing them pain and relieving their suffering.

Christianity: Among the many branches of Christianity, the strongest teachings about diet come within the Seventh-day

Adventist Church. The importance of the health-related data derived from this group has been presented several times earlier. Founder Ellen White was a vegetarian, and lacto-ovo-vegetarianism is officially promoted.[10] Research on followers of this religion has been helpful in demonstrating better health and lifespan in those adhering to plant-based diets. There are groups of scholars that maintain Jesus was a vegetarian.[11]

Islam: Vegetarianism among Muslims is an active movement stressing kindness, mercy, and compassion for animals.[12] The mainstream Muslims who eat meat often follow laws called *halal*, which allow "clean" animals that are properly slaughtered. Certain animals are not permitted, depending on how they are killed, and pork is also forbidden.

Hinduism: There is a strong tradition of vegetarianism in the Hindu religions stemming from the Krishna path and the reverence for the sacred cow. Vegetarianism is viewed as a daily *sadhana*, or spiritual practice, by many Hindus.

Buddhism: There is a strong tradition of vegetarianism among many Buddhists, and Mahayana monks are strict followers, as are many lay practitioners.[13]

Jainism: Originating about the same time as the Hindu and Buddhist religions, Jainism stresses the practice of *ahimsa*, or nonviolence and noninjury.[14] Jains believe in abstaining from meat and honey, and harming any living creature—even insects—is avoided.

Whatever basis forms your path toward whole-food and plant-based meals, you will share a strong tradition with many ethically concerned individuals. In the words of Albert Einstein, "Nothing will benefit human health and increase the chances for survival of life on earth as much as the evolution to a vegetarian diet."[15]

Plant Rant

There is no justification for what goes on behind the closed doors of CAFOs. In fact, Paul McCartney is quoted as saying, "If slaughter-houses had glass walls, everyone would be vegetarian."[16] Or perhaps most everyone—sadly, some people just do not care.

Do humans have domain over animals even if they are boiled, skinned, branded, and cut while alive? In debates of the health attributes of plant-based versus other diets like the LCHF, Paleo, Atkins, and even MED diet, the ethics of raising animals for food is rarely brought up because there simply is no ethical response to the issue of animal mistreatment. Many of the pro-meat experts hide behind the terms "grass-fed," "free-range," and "cage-free," even though these labels often fall short of ensuring that the animals are treated with kindness.

Leading a life based on ahimsa, the Sanskrit word for nonviolence and compassion, can add nobility and purpose at any age. A Sanskrit phrase, heard mainly in yoga studios, is also worth learning: *Lokah samastah sukhino bhavantu* means "May all beings be happy and free, and may the thoughts, words, and actions of my own life contribute in some way to that happiness and to that freedom for all." That is what the Plant-Based Solution can offer to elevate a life to further meaning and purpose, starting with your journey on your new eating plan.

THE PLANT-BASED PLAN   **Learn about the Animal-Rights Movement**

- Watch Gary Yourofsky's free video "The Best Speech You Will Ever Hear" or any of his other videos available on Gary's website, adaptt.org, which is rich in resources for eating and living a plant-based life.

- Become a member of People for the Ethical Treatment of Animals (PETA) or sign up for its newsletter: peta.org.

14

The Earthen Plate
and the Environment

What do the United Nations, Oxford University, and the USDA have in common? They all state that veganism is the answer to our planetary woes. Although this opinion is not based on the ethical treatment of animals, the conclusion is the same: they call for a drastic reduction in diets with animal products and replacing them with plant-based choices for the well-being of the planet. Seeing videos of animals abused is disturbing. Try viewing photos of oceans being polluted, forests being destroyed, and deserts expanding as topsoil blows away. The careful analyses by the UN and other venerated agencies require consideration for how we are going to lead our lives and feed our families.

CASE STUDY
The Amazon Rainforest

Let us turn now to one of the gems of our planet, the Amazon rainforest. This immense expanse of forest, plant life, and animal habitats—over 1 billion acres in five countries—has been untouched for centuries, but the times they are a changin' in the last three decades. A major concern is that the vital role of the Amazon rainforest will never be recovered.

Twenty percent of the world's oxygen is produced in the Amazon rainforest, and more than half of the world's plants, animals, and insects live there.[1] Numerous familiar food items are from the Amazon rainforest, such as figs, coconuts, avocados, mangos, corn, potatoes, rice, yams, squash, and 3,000 varieties of fruits.[2]

Drugs to treat malaria, glaucoma, leukemia, and other diseases are derived from plants found in the Amazon, yet only a fraction of the plants in this biodiverse region have been tested for active compounds that could be used in modern medicine.[3]

All rainforests are crucial to humanity. But because of extractive industries, infrastructure projects, and other threats, we are losing their immensely important treasures at a rapid rate. In the past forty years, the Amazon rainforest has shrunk more than 18 percent (the size of California) due to illegal logging, soy plantations, and cattle ranching, a main cause of deforestation. Most of the remaining forest—its plants, animals, and people who depend on the forest to survive—are under threat.[4]

How can we permit this to continue? What will the world be like when the Amazon—and all rainforests—are a memory?

The rainforests of Brazil have been hit the hardest by cattle ranching, as Brazil is the largest exporter of beef in the world.[5] China, Russia, Europe, and the United States are the main export markets for this beef. Beef is the most carbon-intensive form of meat production and gives rise to more greenhouse gases than all forms of transportation combined. Efforts have been made to slow this destruction, but legal and illegal clearing of forestlands continues. Change is needed before there are no forests. The answer for the earth is the Plant-Based Solution. ■

Study In-Depth: Reducing Greenhouse Gases Easily

By this point in the book, hopefully you or your family have already decided to switch meat-eating habits to meatless. The impact of shifting meat consumption to "faux" plant-based meats was studied in detail by MorningStar Farms, a manufacturer of meat substitutes.[6] The study found that when an American adult chooses to consume a meatless breakfast, lunch, or dinner rather than one that contains meat, the decreased environmental impact for the meal is on average at least 40 percent. In terms of carbon footprint, a switch to a meatless meal results in a 58 percent, 74 percent, and 77 percent reduction compared to a meat-containing meal for breakfast, lunch, and dinner, respectively. For water use, the reductions are 64 percent, 81 percent, and 84 percent for breakfast, lunch, and dinner. Meatless dinners show the highest amount of environmental savings among all the categories, followed by lunches and then breakfasts, primarily because meat-containing dinners contain more meat than breakfast or lunch, as well as the fact that meatless breakfasts were reported to contain a high proportion of dairy.

The study also revealed that a comparison of substitute veggie meats with beef products results in the most benefits (often in the range of 80 percent or 90 percent reductions), with the results for pork and chicken products ranging from 15 percent to a more than 75 percent improvement. The main driver for environmental impacts takes place in the production of raw materials. Raw materials are responsible for about 50 percent of the carbon footprint of meatless meals and 80 percent of the carbon footprint of meat-containing meals.

The biggest difference between meat and non-meat products happens in producing the feed that the animals consume. Raising animals to feed humans requires growing many more plants than if humans consumed the vegetable material directly. Cut out the middleman! Remember, an overall reduction on average of at least 40 percent in terms of environmental impact occurs when switching away from meat.

<hr>

CASE STUDY
James Cameron and the Environment

A long-time environmental advocate and deep-sea diver, director James Cameron made the change to the Plant-Based Solution to help save the earth. His goal was to lower his carbon footprint. He also realized that it would likely improve his health. He was interviewed about the experience for *Men's Journal*, and the example is profound.[7]

He indicated that "the great thing about this as a solution for climate change—one of a number of solutions that we need—is that it's a win-win. You're going to be healthier, you're going to live longer, you're going to look better. You're going to have fewer zits. You're going to be slimmer. You're going to radiate health. You're going to have a better sex drive. That's what shifting away from meat and dairy does."[8]

Cameron is a fan of the Blue Zones (regions of the world with the most centenarians), the documentary *Forks Over Knives*, and the book *The China Study*, which describes research on nutrition and disease performed by T. Colin Campbell, PhD. He is no fan of the Paleo movement, which does not focus on the health of the planet.

When Cameron speaks publically, he eloquently points out that an entry point to the Plant-Based Solution is the realization that as one of over 7 billion human residents of the planet, extreme pressure on the environment requires a reevaluation of our habits and culture right away. He has reduced his family's contribution to greenhouse gases and waste by at least 50 to 75 percent, an example to be copied. He has also established a plant-based K-12 school, the Muse School, in the Los Angeles valley, which hopefully will be replicated also. ◼

Oxford University Speaks Up for the Planet

The headlines were pretty big when Oxford University chimed in on food choices and the environmental consequences. Having conducted the first study to calculate both health and environmental outcomes, they announced some impressive calculations that would result from a transition to a plant-based diet worldwide.[9] The implications they announced were even larger: up to 8 million lives saved by 2050, up to a two-thirds reduction in greenhouse gas emissions, and health-care-related savings of up to 1.5 trillion US dollars.

The Oxford researchers assessed several dietary patterns for 2050, one a business-as-usual plan, one based on a global dietary guideline, one vegan, and the last one vegetarian. The greatest number of deaths avoided, 8.1 million, would be realized with the vegan dietary pattern. Half of those lives saved would come from avoiding red meat and the other half from increased fruit and vegetables in the diet.

The Oxford University research group also estimated the impact of the four dietary models on food-related emissions. They calculated that vegetarian diets would reduce emissions by 63 percent and that vegan diets would produce a 70 percent decrease. Finally, the Oxford researchers looked at the health-care savings by the proposed diets, with the lowest costs being for those following a vegan diet. The work-related savings for vegan diets could reach as high as $20 trillion, a crazy number from the health benefits of just avoiding eggs, meat, and dairy. The Oxford authors called for increased public and private spending on programs geared to reach maximal health and environmental sustainability with the vegan dietary pattern. Those crazy, radical Oxford University hippies sure do like the Plant-Based Solution.

United Nations Speaks Up for Plants

A panel from the United Nations has analyzed the state of our planet and options for survival if we shift to a vegan world.[10] The report by the United Nations Environment Programme (UNEP) found that moving to a meat- and dairy-free diet is critical to saving the world from climate change, hunger, and lack of fuel. The UNEP panel ranked the main global warming contributory factors and pointed out that animal food production was on par with the consumption of fossil fuels. The panel predicted both will choke off the planet if changes are not made. The growing world population and the growing economy of affluence transitions diets toward more meat and dairy, drives up the amount of land required for livestock farming, and supports the food industry that uses power and resources that are many times greater than what is required for plant-based diets.

The UN report stressed that agriculture accounts for 70 percent of global freshwater consumption, 38 percent of total land use, and 19 percent of the world's greenhouse gas emissions. The amount of greenhouse gas emissions from animal farming and meat and dairy production exceeds that emitted from all forms of transportation, including planes, trains, and automobiles. The chairperson of the UNEP panel said that the key necessity was for developing countries to avoid the dietary pattern of meat- and dairy-rich diets of developed Western countries. That would mean avoiding the growth of Kentucky

Fried Chicken, McDonald's, and Arby's in new international markets. There is a fat chance of that happening. The best I believe we can hope for is to demand that the Western food giants offer more energy-efficient plant-based options. Taco Bell and Chipotle have led the way in this.

USDA Guidelines Advisory Committee: Third One Is a Charm

We return again to the powerful process of the advisory committee in establishing the Dietary Guidelines, as there was much attention given to the environmental impact of our food patterns. "For the first time," as reported in a Forks Over Knives article, "the advisory committee concluded that a diet higher in plant-based foods and lower in animal-based foods was both healthier and better for the environment. Their official recommendations for a healthy dietary pattern put vegetables, fruits, and whole grains at the very top of the list and pushed red and processed meats to the very bottom."[11]

Also for the first time, the USDA guidelines committee included environmental sustainability in its recommendations. They considered that a diet lower in animal foods was also better for our planet and that healthy dietary patterns higher in plant-based foods (vegetables, fruits, whole grains, legumes, nuts, and seeds) and lower in calories and animal-based foods are associated with more favorable environmental outcomes (lower greenhouse gas emissions and more favorable land, water, and energy use) than our current American dietary patterns. Those are pretty strong opinions from a committee formed by the USDA to recommend food policy from 2015 to 2020.

The 571-page document reviewed the evidence for plant-based diets being more favorable to the environment. The advisory committee reviewed fifteen scientific studies that assessed dietary patterns and environmental outcomes between the years 2003 and 2014. The Dietary Guidelines Advisory Committee report states, "Overall, the studies were consistent in showing that higher consumption of animal-based foods was associated with higher estimated environmental impact, whereas consumption of more plant-based foods as part of a less meat-based, or vegetarian-style, dietary pattern was associated with an estimated lower environmental impact. One calorie from beef or milk requires 40 or 14 calories of fuel, respectively, whereas 1 calorie from grains can be obtained from 2.2 calories of fuel."[12] Additionally, the evidence showed that dietary patterns that promote health also promote sustainability.

Unfortunately, as the USDA process moved from committee toward final report, the secretary of agriculture and the secretary of health and human services announced that sustainability would be omitted from the final report. They published a blog indicating they planned to remain within the scope of their mandate in the 1990 National Nutrition Monitoring and Related Research Act to provide nutritional and dietary information and guidelines based on the preponderance of the scientific and medical knowledge but not venture into the impact on the environment.[13] Even with this disappointing shift in policy as the guidelines were finalized, the analysis of the advisory committee, along with the reports from the UN and Oxford University, leave no doubt that meaningful actions can come from choosing the Plant-Based Solution. By changing what you eat, you can change the contract between the human species and the natural world.

A comment is necessary regarding a scientist who was an early proponent of the Paleo movement, Boyd Eaton, MD. Trained as a radiologist, he became interested in paleontology and co-wrote a paper in 1985 for a major medical journal on Paleolithic nutrition that argued that a Paleo diet (vegetables, fruits, nuts, roots, and meats; no dairy and grains) is best suited to our ancient genetic makeup.[14] This spurred others to pursue research and writings on the Paleo diet.[15] In late 2015 at a nutrition conference, Dr. Eaton spoke and surprised many by calling for a meatless version of the Paleo diet.[16] His arguments were that beef and other animal protein were simply not sustainable in terms of the world population and the environmental damage. He recommended a shift to plant-protein sources. How refreshing to hear a prominent nutritional thinker consider more than taste in public recommendations of the overall implications of food choices.

Plant Rant

The soft underbelly of the Paleo and low-carb diet movements is that they stress "healthy meats" like grass-fed and free-range options. These buzz words do not account for the environmental burden of an expanding population eating more and more animal-derived foods. There are many excellent resources like the documentary *Cowspiracy* that provide further insight into the impacts of our food choices on the planet. We have the power to decide nearly 80,000 times in a lifetime whether our meals reflect a concern for the future of the earth. The careful analyses of Oxford, the UN, and the USDA along with other research makes it clear that we must move to plant-based eating and that the impact would be profound.

THE PLANT-BASED PLAN   **Learn How a
Plant-Based Diet Helps the Environment**

Watch the movie *Cowspiracy: The Sustainability Secret* (available on Netflix or for purchase at cowspiracy.com).

A Twenty-One-Day Menu
with Recipes (and Bonus Recipes)

I f you turned to this chapter first, welcome. You do not need to know the science or the compelling case studies to enjoy the dozens of recipes that follow. All you need is a passion for great-tasting food that is relatively easy to make and share with family and friends. You can experiment, make mistakes, make some improvements, and still improve your health and the health of the planet.

This is a journey, so if you make some errors or fall off the wagon, just start again the next day and focus on your "why": better health, pride in helping the environment, and kindness to animals. If you live alone or are a couple, you might want to cut some of the recipes in half. If you are joining the Plant-Based Solution with a family that is not fully supportive or with children who are not on board with the diet, you may have to make two meals for a while like we did until our children were on board (late in their teens, so it was a long period of preparing two meals many evenings).

I am excited to share this twenty-one-day plan with dozens of recipes. A frequent observation is that when people rid themselves of meat, eggs, and dairy and replace them with the flavors, textures, and the dense nutrition of plant-based meals, they have no interest in turning back to old habits that did not promote their health to the fullest. This is where the rubber meets the road without meat.

These recipes have been made in the Kahn kitchen and passed the taste and preparation test by my wife, Karen Kahn, RN, BSN, who is a certified plant-based food educator. You can find fancier recipes, and perhaps you can find simpler ones, but I am confident you can be off to a satisfying and successful start to your plant-based journey if you whip together these meals.

Generally, breakfast is the easiest. If you are tentative, maybe breakfast is the best place to start. Some people like to put their foot into the water for a while before diving in. However, if you are facing medical problems and looking for a proven path to try to reverse them, you should go twenty-one days in a row fully engaged in the Plant-Based Solution.

Day 1

The Plant-Based Plan: Enhance breakfast with fruit. No bowl of cereal or oatmeal should be without adornment by berries, dates, bananas, or raisins. Although dried fruit should be used in moderation, children often will eat it over whole fruit. It's a start.

BREAKFAST   RAW OATS

I love raw oats. I keep a large container in my pantry of this mixture and I leave a ½-cup scoop in the container to scoop out a serving at a time. You can add nuts, berries, bananas, or dried fruit to your bowl of oats too!

INGREDIENTS
- 1 bag (1 pound) rolled oats
  (I use Bob's Red Mill Gluten-Free Rolled Oats.)
- ½ cup cacao nibs
- ½ cup sunflower seeds
- ½ cup pumpkin seeds
- ½ cup goji berries
  Lots of cinnamon
- 1 cup plant milk (rice, almond, soy)
  Toppings of your choice

INSTRUCTIONS

1. Combine the dry ingredients, then store in an airtight container.
2. For each serving, scoop ½ cup of the dry oat mixture into a bowl.
3. Add plant milk and stir well.
4. Add toppings.

LUNCH   MASHED CHICKPEA SALAD

INGREDIENTS

1	can (15 ounces) chickpeas (garbanzo beans), rinsed
½	cup celery, sliced
½	cup carrots, diced
¼–⅓	cup scallions, sliced
¼	cup (or more) hummus or tahini
1–2	tablespoons mustard (stoneground or Dijon)
	Dash of garlic powder
½	teaspoon ground cumin
	Sea salt and freshly ground pepper
	Juice of 1 lemon (optional)
1	small handful of pumpkin seeds (optional)
	Paprika or smoked paprika (garnish)

INSTRUCTIONS

1. Place the chickpeas in a medium bowl and mash roughly with a fork or potato masher.
2. Add the remaining ingredients and mix. If you like a creamier consistency, add more hummus.
3. Taste for seasoning.
4. Sprinkle with paprika and serve however you like—make a sandwich, serve on a bed of leafy greens, or scoop up with crackers or sliced vegetables, such as cucumbers, bell peppers, and celery sticks.

Note: If your hummus is a bit thick, thin it out with a tablespoon or two of water. Store leftovers in an airtight container in the fridge for up to a week. I make sandwiches with this when we travel.

DINNER   EASY THREE-BEAN CHILI

INGREDIENTS

1	small onion, diced
2	carrots, diced
1	cup water or vegetable broth
1	can (15 ounces) diced tomatoes
1	can (15 ounces) chickpeas, drained
1	can (15 ounces) cannellini beans, drained
1	can (15 ounces) kidney beans, drained
4	ounces frozen corn
1	garlic clove, minced
1	tablespoon chili powder
1	teaspoon ground cumin
1	teaspoon oregano
1	teaspoon basil
½	teaspoon sugar

INSTRUCTIONS

1. Sauté the onion and carrots in ½ cup water in a large saucepan.
2. Stir in the tomatoes. Cook for a few minutes.
3. Add the rest of the water.
4. Add the beans, corn, garlic, spices, and sugar.
5. Cover and simmer for 20 minutes.

Note: Add leftover spinach or kale and/or top with cooked brown rice or quinoa.

Day 2

The Plant-Based Plan: Buy a glass or stainless water bottle and fill it every morning with fresh water. I would strongly recommend a home water-treatment system. You can stop buying bottled water and the plastics that leach into the water. Add a slice of cucumber, a sprig of mint, or a slice of lemon or lime.

BREAKFAST   GREEN SMOOTHIE

INGREDIENTS

½   cup rolled oats

½   cup frozen spinach

½   cup frozen mango

1   banana

½   lime, peeled (or just the juice)

2   tablespoons hemp seeds

1   tablespoon peanut butter

1   cup unsweetened almond milk or other plant milk

Water (about ½ to 1 cup, for desired consistency)

INSTRUCTIONS

1. Blend all the ingredients.
2. Add more liquid if needed.

LUNCH   LOADED SWEET POTATO

INGREDIENTS

2   medium sweet potatoes

1   garlic clove, minced

Splash of vegetable broth for sautéing

1   bunch of kale, washed, destemmed, and torn into pieces

1   can (15 ounces) black beans, drained and rinsed

Sea salt and freshly ground pepper

Salsa (optional)

INSTRUCTIONS

1. Preheat the oven to 375 degrees.
2. Pierce the potatoes a few times with a fork and place them in the oven on a tray with parchment paper. (In case the potatoes leak, your oven stays clean.)
3. Bake the potatoes for 45 minutes or until cooked through.
4. Meanwhile, sauté the garlic in broth.

5. Add the kale to the garlic. Cover and cook for a few minutes.
6. Add the beans and cook for a few minutes. Season to taste.
7. Cut the potatoes in half lengthwise. Top with the bean and kale mixture.
8. Top with salsa if desired.

DINNER   LENTIL LOAF

This recipe is adapted from *Prevent and Reverse Heart Disease* by Dr. Caldwell Esselstyn. Ruth Kahn makes this, and it is delicious.

INGREDIENTS

2   medium onions, diced

1   garlic clove, minced

6   mushrooms, chopped

   Splash of vegetable broth or water for sautéing

2   cups fresh spinach, chopped

1   package (8 ounces) of precooked lentils (or drained, canned lentils), mashed with a fork (see note)

2   cups rolled oats

1   cup brown rice, cooked

1   can (15 ounces) diced tomatoes, drained

2   teaspoons thyme

1½   teaspoons rosemary

GLAZE

3   tablespoons ketchup

1   tablespoon balsamic vinegar

1   tablespoon maple syrup

INSTRUCTIONS

1. Preheat the oven to 350 degrees.
2. Sauté the onions, garlic, and mushrooms in the broth. When they soften, add the spinach.

3. Stir in the lentils, oats, rice, tomatoes, and herbs.
4. Prepare a baking sheet with parchment paper.
5. Form a loaf with your hands.
6. Mix the glaze and brush it on top of the loaf.
7. Bake for 45 to 60 minutes. Cool slightly before serving.

Note: Precooked lentils are usually located in the produce section—refrigerated and packaged in a plastic bag. Slice a piece of the loaf for a tasty sandwich for lunch.

Day 3

The Plant-Based Plan: Throw a handful of any greens you have on hand into as many meals as possible during the last few minutes of cooking.

BREAKFAST   BLUEBERRY APPLE OATS

INGREDIENTS
- ½ cup frozen or fresh blueberries
- 1 small apple, grated
- ½ cup rolled oats
- 1 cup plant milk
- Toppings of your choice: nuts, seeds, fresh or dried fruit (optional)

INSTRUCTIONS
1. Place the blueberries in a saucepan with a splash of hot water. Let them cook for 5 minutes until the blueberries are soft and juicy. Pour them into a glass bowl.
2. Mix the apple, oats, and milk in the saucepan and cook for 3 to 5 minutes, until hot and creamy.
3. Add the oat mixture into the blueberries and stir.
4. Serve with optional toppings.

LUNCH HEARTY SPLIT PEA SOUP

INGREDIENTS

2   garlic cloves, minced

1   onion, diced (see note)

8   cups water (or 4 cups water and 4 cups broth)

2   cups dried green split peas, rinsed

2   stalks celery, diced

2   large carrots, diced

1   medium potato (or sweet potato), diced

½   teaspoon basil

½   teaspoon thyme

Sea salt and freshly ground pepper

1   bay leaf

A few handfuls of spinach (optional)

INSTRUCTIONS

1. In a large pot, sauté the garlic and onion in a little of the water for a few minutes.
2. Add the rest of the water and add the peas.
3. Cover and simmer for about 30 minutes.
4. Add the remaining ingredients. Cook another 30 minutes.
5. Let the soup cool. Remove the bay leaf. Use an immersion blender to make the soup the consistency you choose.
6. Throw in some optional spinach to increase your greens.

Note: To save time, use a prepackaged mirepoix mix (chopped onions, celery, and carrots). Sauté the mix with the garlic in step 1, then add the potato and spices in step 4.

DINNER   KALE AND SWEET POTATO SALAD WITH DRIED CRANBERRIES

Recipe by Darshana Thacker, courtesy of Forks Over Knives.

This simple kale salad recipe delivers big on flavor. Steamed sweet potatoes, cranberries, and cashews bring an array of colors and textures. The dressing gets its creamy texture and smoky-sweet flavor from a combination of tahini and smoked paprika.

INGREDIENTS

- 1 medium sweet potato, cut into ¾-inch dice (about 3 cups)
- 6 ounces kale, shredded (6 cups)
- ½ cup dried cranberries
- 2 tablespoons chopped cashews
- 2 tablespoons finely chopped fresh parsley

DRESSING

- 2 tablespoons tahini
- 2 tablespoons lemon juice
- 2 teaspoons smoked paprika
- ½ teaspoon fresh garlic, minced (1 clove)
- Sea salt and freshly ground black pepper

INSTRUCTIONS

1. Place a steamer insert in a saucepan over 1 to 2 inches of water. Bring water to a boil, add sweet potatoes, cover, and steam for about 20 minutes, until potatoes are very tender when pierced with a sharp knife. Transfer potatoes to a large bowl to cool.

2. To make the dressing, combine the tahini, lemon juice, smoked paprika, garlic, and ½ cup water in a glass jar. Cover jar with a tight-fitting lid and shake well to blend the ingredients. Taste the dressing, add salt and pepper to taste, and shake again.

3. In a large salad bowl, combine the sweet potatoes, kale, cranberries, cashews, and parsley. Pour the dressing over the salad and mix well. For best results, let the salad stand for 15 to 20 minutes before serving.

Day 4

The Plant-Based Plan: Make sure you eat foods rich in beta-carotene and the family called carotenoids every day. These include dark leafy greens like kale and collard greens, sweet potatoes, carrots, and red and orange peppers. Your skin and immune system will thank you.

BREAKFAST   POTATO HASH

INGREDIENTS

- 3   medium potatoes, peeled and cubed
- 1   large sweet potato, peeled and cubed
- 1   onion, sliced
- 1   teaspoon fresh thyme
- 1   teaspoon sea salt
- 1   teaspoon freshly ground pepper
- 1   handful of spinach

FOR THE SKILLET

- 1   small onion, chopped
- 2   cloves garlic, minced
- ¼   cup vegetable broth or water
- Sea salt and freshly ground pepper to taste

INSTRUCTIONS

1. Mix the potato cubes with the onion and seasonings. Spread on a tray lined with parchment paper. Bake at 400 degrees for about 40 minutes. Stir after 20 minutes.
2. In a skillet, sauté the onion and garlic in broth or water. Cook for about 4 to 6 minutes.
3. Remove the potatoes from the oven, and stir them into the skillet. Add the spinach. Cook for a few minutes.
4. Adjust seasonings to taste.

Note: You can get creative by adding leftover beans, tempeh, mushrooms, and other vegetables.

LUNCH VEGGIE REUBEN WITH CASHEW CHEESE

Recipe by VeggieChick.com.

INGREDIENTS

CASHEW CHEESE

¾ cup raw cashews (if not using high-powered blender, soak overnight in water and drain)

1 tablespoon nutritional yeast

¼ teaspoon garlic powder

2 teaspoons tahini

1 tablespoon Dijon mustard

2 tablespoons lemon juice

¼ cup water

TOPPINGS

10 ounces sauerkraut, drained

Basil leaves

Spinach leaves

Tomato slices

8 slices pumpernickel bread or gluten-free bread if desired

Vegan butter

INSTRUCTIONS

1. Make the cashew cheese. In a high-powered blender or food processor, add the cashews, nutritional yeast, and garlic powder. Process until blended into a fine powder. Add the tahini, Dijon mustard, and water, and blend until smooth. (If using soaked cashews, add with all cheese ingredients.)

2. Make the sandwiches. Place a skillet over medium heat for 5 minutes. Spread a little vegan butter on 2 pieces of pumpernickel bread. In the pan, add 1 piece of bread (butter side down), and then spread 1 to 2 tablespoons of the cashew cheese on the bread. Add a few pieces of spinach, 1 to 2 tablespoons of sauerkraut, a slice of tomato, and a couple leaves of basil.

3. Top with remaining piece of bread (buttered side up) and carefully flatten with a large spatula.

4. Cover and heat for about 4 minutes, and then flip and cook another 4 minutes, or until bread is crispy on each side and sandwich is warm. Cut in half and serve.

DINNER   KIDNEY BEAN AND LENTIL DAL

Recipe by Darshana Thacker, courtesy of Forks Over Knives.

This kidney bean and lentil dal is a staple in every home in north India and is also found on the menu in every Indian restaurant serving north Indian food. It gets its strong aromatic flavor from ginger, garlic, coriander, turmeric, and other warming spices. Serve with any cooked grain or whole-grain bread or tortillas.

INGREDIENTS

¼   medium red onion, cut into ¼-inch dice (about ½ cup)

3   cloves garlic, minced (1½ teaspoons)

1   teaspoon grated fresh gingerroot

1   tomato, cut into ¼-inch dice (about 1 cup)

2   teaspoons ground coriander

½   teaspoon ground turmeric

¼   teaspoon ground cloves

¼   teaspoon ground cinnamon

1   teaspoon ground cumin

1   cup unsweetened, unflavored plant milk

1   can (15 ounces) brown lentils, drained and rinsed (or 1½ cups cooked)

1   can (15 ounces) red kidney beans, drained and rinsed (or 1½ cups cooked)

1   tablespoon fresh lime juice
    Sea salt

1   tablespoon fresh cilantro, finely chopped
    Brown rice, whole-grain bread, or tortillas (for serving)

INSTRUCTIONS

1. Combine the onions, garlic, ginger, and ¼ cup water in a nonstick saucepan and cook over medium-low heat, stirring occasionally, until the onions start to turn golden brown, about 10 minutes.
2. Add the tomato, coriander, turmeric, cloves, cinnamon, and cumin; mix well. Add ½ cup water and cook until the tomatoes are cooked through, 5 to 7 minutes.
3. Add the plant milk, lentils, and beans and continue to cook until the dal thickens, 5 to 10 minutes.
4. Add the lime juice. Mix well, and then season with salt to taste. Cook until the flavors merge, 2 minutes.
5. Garnish with cilantro.
6. Serve hot with brown rice, bread, or tortillas.

Day 5

The Plant-Based Plan: Buy several bags of frozen berries for your freezer. Having them handy makes it easy to add berries to your cereal, smoothie, muffins, or breads. Berries are low in plant sugar and very high in nutrients. They are very good for the heart and brain.

BREAKFAST   FRENCH TOAST

INGREDIENTS

1   cup plant milk
1   tablespoon maple syrup
2   tablespoons flour
1   tablespoon nutritional yeast
1   teaspoon cinnamon
¼   teaspoon nutmeg
1   teaspoon vanilla extract
    Pinch of sea salt
6   slices of day-old bread
    Maple syrup and fruit (for serving)

INSTRUCTIONS

1. In a small bowl, combine the milk, maple syrup, flour, nutritional yeast, cinnamon, nutmeg, vanilla, and salt.
2. Place a few slices of the bread in a 9-by-9-inch glass dish. Pour the mixture over the bread.
3. Move the bread around to coat, and flip the bread over.
4. Heat a large skillet over medium heat. Cook the coated bread until both sides are golden brown.
5. Serve the French toast with maple syrup and fruit.

LUNCH   WATERCRESS SALAD

Our daughter-in-law, Yanelys, makes this delicious salad. There is never any left over!

INGREDIENTS

1	bag watercress, shredded
	Juice of 1 lemon
½	cup cilantro, chopped
½	medium onion, diced
2	tablespoons extra-virgin olive oil
1	avocado, sliced
1	can (15 ounces) hearts of palm, sliced
1	tomato, sliced
	Pinch of salt

INSTRUCTIONS

1. Wash the watercress in a bowl of water with ¼ teaspoon of vinegar.
2. Combine all the ingredients.
3. Mix well and serve.

DINNER   EASY BLACK BEAN BURGERS

INGREDIENTS

- 1   prepackaged mirepoix (16 ounces)
    (or 1 onion, 2 carrots, 3 celery stalks, chopped)
- 1   garlic clove, minced
    Splash of vegetable broth for sautéing
- 1   handful of spinach
- 1   sweet potato, cubed and cooked
- 1   can (15 ounces) black beans, drained
- 1   cup rolled oats
- 1   teaspoon ground cumin
- 1   teaspoon chili powder
- ¼   teaspoon cayenne pepper
    Buns and burger toppings (for serving)

INSTRUCTIONS

1. Preheat the oven to 350 degrees.
2. Sauté the mirepoix and garlic in vegetable broth over medium heat. Add the spinach.
3. Process the mirepoix, potato, and beans in a food processor until smooth.
4. Add the oats, cumin, chili powder, and pepper, and process until mixed.
5. Put the burger mixture in a bowl in the refrigerator while you clean up.
6. Line a baking tray with parchment paper.
7. Form the patties and place on the parchment paper.
8. Bake for about 20 minutes. Patties should be firm.
    Flip with a spatula and bake another 10 minutes or so.
9. Serve on toasted buns with toppings.

Note: These burgers freeze well. Just reheat and serve.

Day 6

The Plant-Based Plan: Make it a habit to eat a small amount of raw nuts daily, but no more than a small handful. Mix walnuts, Brazil nuts, almonds, and hazelnuts and store in a glass jar. Add a few to cereal, salads, or on casseroles.

BREAKFAST   TOFU SCRAMBLE

INGREDIENTS

1	block firm tofu, pressed between two plates to drain the water
1	tablespoon tamari
1	tablespoon nutritional yeast
1–2	garlic cloves, minced
½	tablespoon turmeric
½	tablespoon black pepper
¼	tablespoon ground cumin
	Chopped veggies: red pepper, onion, mushrooms, spinach, or any others you have left in the fridge

INSTRUCTIONS

1. Crumble the tofu with your hands or mash with a fork in a bowl.
2. Add all the other ingredients, and mix together well.
3. Transfer the tofu mixture to a skillet and cook over medium heat.
4. Stir and cook until the liquid evaporates.

Note: This is an easy recipe that you can modify by changing the vegetables. You can add beans and mix with salsa, for example.

LUNCH   WILD RICE AND GREENS

INGREDIENTS

- 1   cup wild rice
- 4   cups water
- 5   ounces greens (arugula, spinach, or a mixture)
- 1   can (15 ounces) of your favorite beans, rinsed
- 2   stalks of celery, chopped
- 1   carrot, shredded
- ½   cup toasted nuts or seeds of choice

DRESSING

- 3   tablespoons balsamic vinegar
- 1   tablespoon maple syrup
- 2   teaspoons Dijon mustard
- Sea salt and freshly ground pepper

INSTRUCTIONS

1. Cook the rice in the water over medium heat. Simmer covered for about 35 minutes, until tender.
2. Place the rice in a strainer and rinse with cool water.
3. Toss the rice, greens, beans, celery, carrot, and nuts or seeds together.
4. Combine the dressing ingredients. Toss with the rice and vegetables. Season with salt and pepper.

DINNER   VEGGIE LASAGNA

INGREDIENTS

- 1   onion, chopped
- 2   garlic cloves, minced
- 2   handfuls of fresh spinach
- 1   cup sautéed mixed veggies of choice
- Splash of vegetable broth
- 1   can (15 ounces) cannellini beans, rinsed and mashed
- 1   jar (26 ounces) marinara sauce (oil-free, if possible)

6 gluten-free lasagna noodles

2 tablespoons nutritional yeast

INSTRUCTIONS

1. Preheat the oven to 350 degrees.
2. Sauté the onion, garlic, spinach, and other veggies for a few minutes in the broth.
3. Combine the veggies and beans (by hand or in a food processor).
4. Pour a little of the marinara in a baking dish. Lay three lasagna noodles on top.
5. Spread half of the vegetable and bean mixture on top of the noodles, and cover with more sauce.
6. Lay 3 more noodles on top. Spread the rest of the veggie mixture on the noodles, top with sauce, and sprinkle nutritional yeast over the lasagna.
7. Bake for 35 to 45 minutes.

Day 7

The Plant-Based Plan: Learn to read labels and buy bread that is 100 percent whole grain. Some varieties have seeds added for more fiber. They are delicious. Pay attention to the sodium content of store-bought bread. Even those that say "100 percent whole wheat" may be high in sodium, so comparison shop to buy the brands that are lower in sodium.

BREAKFAST   GRILLED NUT BUTTER AND APPLE SANDWICH

INGREDIENTS

Almond butter

4 slices of bread

2 apples, sliced into long pieces

Cinnamon

Maple syrup

Oil spray

INSTRUCTIONS

1. Add a layer of nut butter to all 4 slices of bread.
2. Layer 2 slices of the bread with apples. Sprinkle with cinnamon, and add a light drizzle of maple syrup over the top. Set aside any remaining apple slices.
3. Top layered bread with the other slices of bread.
4. Grease a skillet with oil spray and heat over medium. Place sandwich in skillet, and cook for about 2 to 4 minutes.
5. Flip and cook another 2 to 4 minutes. Remove from heat and serve with any remaining apple slices on the side.

LUNCH   POTATO SPINACH BEAN CURRY

INGREDIENTS

- 2   potatoes, cubed
- 1   can (8 ounces) light coconut milk
- 3   carrots, sliced
- 1   can (15 ounces) diced tomatoes
- 1½   teaspoons turmeric
- 1½   teaspoons ground cumin
- 1   teaspoon red pepper flakes
  Sea salt and freshly ground pepper
- 1   can (15 ounces) cannellini beans, rinsed
- 4   ounces spinach
  Cooked rice or quinoa (see note) (for serving)

INSTRUCTIONS

1. Cook the potatoes in a pot of water until tender. Drain.
2. Add to the potatoes the coconut milk, carrots, tomatoes, spices, and salt and pepper. Cover and simmer for about 30 minutes, until carrots are soft.
3. Add the beans and spinach. Cover and let the residual heat warm the beans and wilt the spinach.
4. Serve over rice or quinoa.

Note: Use leftover grains or frozen or precooked packaged rice.

DINNER CAULIFLOWER PURÉE WITH SAUTÉED MUSHROOMS

Recipe by VeggieChick.com.

INGREDIENTS

1   head cauliflower, broken into florets
1   tablespoon nutritional yeast
½   teaspoon sea salt
¼   teaspoon black pepper
2   garlic cloves, minced
½   cup unsweetened almond milk
1   cup unsalted vegetable broth
1   large shallot, chopped fine (about ⅓ cup)
2   cups cremini or white mushrooms, halved
½   tablespoon tamari (or soy sauce)
½   teaspoon garlic powder
2   cups chopped Swiss chard
    Juice of 1 lemon

INSTRUCTIONS

1. Boil cauliflower until soft, about 7 to 8 minutes.
2. Drain, rinse, and add cauliflower to high-powered blender or food processor. Add nutritional yeast, salt, pepper, garlic, and almond milk. Blend until smooth.
3. In a large skillet, add the broth over medium-high heat. Add the shallots and mushrooms. Cook for 10 minutes, stirring occasionally until mushrooms are soft. Add tamari, garlic powder, and Swiss chard. Stir about 1 minute until the Swiss chard is wilted.
4. Remove from heat. In a bowl, add cauliflower purée and top with mushroom–Swiss chard mix. Drizzle with lemon juice. Makes 4 small servings. Serve with salad or bread.

Note: This dish will last for 1 to 2 days in the fridge but is best served fresh.

Day 8

The Plant-Based Plan: Fill a glass jar with ground flax seed, chia seeds, and hemp seeds. Use this seed mixture on your cereal, oatmeal, and in a smoothie every day to add fiber and healthy, plant-based omega-3 fatty acids to your diet.

BREAKFAST OVERNIGHT OATS

INGREDIENTS

- ½ cup rolled oats
- ⅔ cup plant milk
- ½ teaspoon vanilla extract
  Dash maple syrup (optional)
  Toppings of your choice: cinnamon, raisins, nuts, fruit (for serving)

INSTRUCTIONS

1. Combine all the ingredients together in small bowl.
2. Let it sit covered in the refrigerator overnight.
3. Serve with toppings.

Note: I use small glass bowls that come with lids. I make several individual servings at a time and stack them on the top shelf of the refrigerator. Get creative. I often add apple butter, nut butter, or a fruit jam to the oatmeal.

LUNCH QUINOA HARVEST BOWL

INGREDIENTS

- 1 cup Brussels sprouts, sliced in half
  Splash of vegetable broth
- 1 cup arugula
- ½ cup cooked quinoa
- 1 tablespoon pumpkin seeds
- ½ avocado, sliced
  Sea salt and freshly ground pepper

TAHINI-MISO DRESSING

- ¼ cup tahini
- 1 tablespoon miso
- 1 tablespoon lemon juice
- ¼ cup or more warm water
- ¼ teaspoon freshly ground pepper

INSTRUCTIONS

1. Sauté the Brussels sprouts in the broth for about 15 minutes.
2. Arrange the arugula, quinoa, and Brussels sprouts in a bowl.
3. Place the seeds and avocado on top. Season to taste.
4. Combine the dressing ingredients in a separate bowl and mix well.
5. Drizzle the dressing over the quinoa.

DINNER BUTTERNUT SQUASH SPINACH BOWL

INGREDIENTS

- 1 cup short-grain brown rice
- 2 cups water or vegetable broth (or combination)
- 1 small butternut squash, diced (about 2½ cups; you can find pre-cut squash at Trader Joe's)
- 1 tablespoon olive oil
- ½ teaspoon thyme (rub it between your palms when you sprinkle over the squash)
  Sea salt to taste
- 1 small onion, chopped
- 1 teaspoon garlic, minced
- 2–3 handfuls baby spinach
- 1 can (15 ounces) cannellini or your favorite beans, drained and rinsed
  Sea salt and freshly ground pepper, to taste

INSTRUCTIONS

1. Preheat the oven to 400 degrees.
2. In a medium pot, add rice and water, bring to a boil, cover, reduce heat to low, and simmer for 30 minutes.

3. Remove cover and let rest for 5 to 10 minutes. Fluff with a fork.

4. While the rice is simmering, place squash on a roasting pan lined with parchment paper. Toss the squash in olive oil and sprinkle with the thyme and salt. Place on middle rack and bake for 25 to 30 minutes, stirring once. Pierce it with a fork to see if it is tender.

5. In a medium pan over medium heat, add a splash of vegetable broth, add onions and garlic, and cook for about 5 minutes. Add spinach and cook until wilted. Add beans and cook until heated through.

Day 9

The Plant-Based Plan: Put brightly colored fruits in a bowl on the counter. They will be gone in place of cookies and crackers. Plan two trips to the produce market each week to keep the fruit bowl refilled.

BREAKFAST APPLE-CINNAMON OATMEAL BOWL

INGREDIENTS

1 small apple, chopped

2 tablespoons walnuts, chopped

¼ teaspoon pumpkin pie spice

¼ teaspoon cinnamon

1½ cups water

¾ cup rolled oats

Pinch of sea salt

1 tablespoon ground flax seeds

2 tablespoons raisins

1 tablespoon brown sugar

Splash of almond milk

Toppings such as brown sugar, walnuts, raisins, and fresh apple slices (for serving)

INSTRUCTIONS

1. In a small saucepan, combine the apple with a little water over medium heat. Sauté for 2 minutes.
2. Add the walnuts, pumpkin pie spice, and cinnamon to the pan. Stir and toast for 1 minute.
3. Add the water and bring to a boil.
4. Add the oats and salt. Turn the heat down to medium-low and simmer until the oats begin to thicken.
5. Add the flax seeds (this will help thicken the oatmeal), raisins, brown sugar, and almond milk. Cook until thick.
6. Serve with toppings.

LUNCH BLACK BEAN ENCHILADAS

INGREDIENTS

SMOKY BLACK BEANS

1	can (15 ounces) black beans
1	garlic clove, minced
¼	cup water
½	teaspoon coriander
½	teaspoon ground cumin
¼	teaspoon smoked paprika
¼	teaspoon sea salt

ENCHILADA SAUCE

2	tablespoons extra-virgin olive oil
1½	tablespoons flour
1	teaspoon garlic powder
1	tablespoon oregano
3	tablespoons chili powder
2	teaspoons ground cumin
½	teaspoon sea salt
	Pinch of cinnamon

2   tablespoons tomato paste

1   cup vegetable broth

1   teaspoon apple cider vinegar

FILLING

1   small onion, chopped

Pinch of sea salt

Splash of vegetable broth

1   red pepper, seeded and chopped

1   teaspoon ground cumin

¼   teaspoon cinnamon

4   ounces fresh spinach

Corn tortillas

INSTRUCTIONS

1. Preheat the oven to 400 degrees.
2. Make the smoky black beans: Put all the ingredients in a medium saucepan and cook for 5 to 8 minutes. Set aside.
3. Make the enchilada sauce: Heat the oil, and then add the flour. Whisk. Add the spices and tomato paste. Slowly add the broth. Stir for a few minutes. Let the sauce cook and thicken. Remove it from the heat when it thickens. Add the vinegar. Set aside.
4. Make the filling: Sauté the onion and salt in the broth over medium heat. Add the red pepper and sauté until the veggies soften. Add the cumin and cinnamon. Add the spinach and cook until wilted. Remove from the heat. Stir the smoky black beans into the filling and add a few tablespoons of the sauce.
5. Assemble the enchiladas: Pour ¼ cup of sauce in a 9-by-13-inch pan. Tilt to spread the sauce around. Put ½ cup of the filling on a tortilla, roll up the sides, and then roll up the middle. Place the seam down in the pan. Repeat. Cover the enchiladas with sauce.
6. Bake 20 minutes.

DINNER BAKED VEGETABLE POLENTA

INGREDIENTS

- 2 cups or more of water
- 1 cup ground organic cornmeal
- ½ teaspoon thyme
- 1 cup corn (fresh or frozen)
- 1 clove garlic, minced
  Pinch of sea salt
- 2 cups sliced mushrooms (white button mushrooms are inexpensive and work well)
- 2 cups kale, washed, de-stemmed, and chopped
- ½ cup nutritional yeast (great source of vitamin B12)
  Sea salt and freshly ground pepper to taste

INSTRUCTIONS

1. Preheat the oven to 350 degrees.
2. Bring 2 cups of water to boil. Add the cornmeal and stir with a wooden spoon to prevent clumps.
3. Add the corn and thyme. Turn down the heat and cook for about 10 minutes. If it gets too thick, add a little water.
4. Spray a large skillet with cooking oil or use a splash of vegetable broth. Add the garlic and mushrooms.
5. Add a pinch of salt. Stir until the mushrooms begin to give off liquid.
6. Add the kale and another tablespoon of water. Stir and let cook for about a minute.
7. Add the kale and mushroom mixture to the cornmeal.
8. Add the nutritional yeast and stir to combine.
9. Pour the mixture into a glass baking dish. Bake for 15 minutes. Let cool and cut into squares.

Note: This is also delicious with marinara sauce. And it makes great leftovers.

Day 10

The Plant-Based Plan: Cooking with beans is a habit you want to make part of your health habits. If you use canned beans, look for brands that say BPA-free. Rinse the beans well. Store unused portions in the refrigerator to make them easy to add to a salad, into soup, and even hidden in muffins and brownies. Beans are rich in fiber and are a Blue Zone food (see chapter 12) associated with longevity.

BREAKFAST   CHICKPEA OMELET

INGREDIENTS

- 1 cup chickpea flour
- ¾–1 cup plant milk
- 2–3 tablespoons nutritional yeast
- ½ teaspoon baking powder
- ¼ teaspoon turmeric
- Sea salt and freshly ground pepper
- Chopped veggies of your choice (Use up what is left in your veggie drawer.)
- Splash of vegetable broth
- Vegan cheese, shredded (optional)

INSTRUCTIONS

1. Make the batter by combining all the ingredients except the veggies, broth, and cheese. Mix well and set aside.
2. Lightly sauté the veggies in the broth.
3. Pour the batter on top of the veggies and cover. Cook for a few minutes.
4. Flip the omelet.
5. Sprinkle with shredded cheese.

LUNCH   MAKE A BUDDHA BOWL

It's so easy to make a Buddha Bowl. Be creative and use what's in the house or try something new!

FOR THE BOWL

GREENS
1 cup of greens of choice, such as arugula, kale, spinach, or combo

GRAINS
1 cup of grains, such as rice, quinoa, millet, or barley

PROTEIN
1 cup of beans of choice or lentils, tofu, or edamame

VEGGIES
Chopped veggies of choice, raw or steamed

NUTS, SEEDS, AVOCADO
Add sliced avocado. Sprinkle with nuts or seeds.

DRESSING
Vinegar, miso-tahini, or peanut butter

MAKE A DRESSING

VINEGAR
Mix ⅓ cup balsamic or apple cider vinegar with 1 tablespoon mustard of choice and 1 teaspoon of maple syrup.

MISO-TAHINI
Combine ⅓ cup tahini, 1 tablespoon miso paste, 1 teaspoon lemon juice, 1 teaspoon maple syrup, and crushed garlic (optional) to taste.

PEANUT-MISO
Combine 2 tablespoons peanut butter, 1 tablespoon miso paste, 1 tablespoon maple syrup, ½ cup water, and 1 to 2 teaspoons of tamari.

INSTRUCTIONS
1. Layer the ingredients in a bowl. Drizzle with dressing.

DINNER CURRIED GNOCCHI WITH GOLDEN BEETS

Recipe by VeggieChick.com.

INGREDIENTS

2 cups plus 2 tablespoons unsalted vegetable broth

3 garlic cloves, minced

1 white onion, diced

1 medium golden beet, peeled and cut into 1-inch slices (about 2 cups)

3 cups Swiss chard (remove white parts)

1 teaspoon ground coriander

1 teaspoon curry powder

½ teaspoon cumin

½ teaspoon sea salt

1 17-ounce package gnocchi

INSTRUCTIONS

1. Heat a large skillet over medium-high heat. Add 2 tablespoons of broth. Add garlic and cook for 1 minute, being careful not to burn. Add onion and cook 1 minute, stirring. Add beets and cook for 3 minutes. Add Swiss chard, remaining 2 cups vegetable broth, and the spices.

2. Cover and reduce heat to medium. Simmer for about 8 to 9 minutes or until beets are tender. Add gnocchi to mixture, cover, and simmer for 3 to 4 minutes.

3. Remove from heat and serve. Add salt to taste.

Day 11

The Plant-Based Plan: A resource to find quality and non-GMO dry goods is ThriveMarket.com. Thousands of name-brand food items and products—like those found in a big box store, which you may not have locally—can be shipped to your porch in small quantities. Plus, the prices are lower than at most of those stores.

BREAKFAST   DIY MUESLI

INGREDIENTS

1½   cups rolled oats

½   cup raw pumpkin seeds

½   cup raw almonds or other nut of choice

½   cup raw sunflower seeds

3   tablespoons hemp seeds

2   tablespoons chia seeds

¼   cup dried fruit, such as raisins, cranberries, or goji berries

½   teaspoon ground cinnamon

Plant milk, fresh berries, sliced banana (for serving)

INSTRUCTIONS

1. Preheat the oven to 325 degrees.
2. Place the oats, seeds, and nuts on a baking tray lined with parchment paper, and bake for 10 to 15 minutes. Stir every few minutes so they do not burn.
3. Remove from the oven and cool. Transfer to a bowl.
4. Add the remaining ingredients to the bowl and stir well.
5. Scoop out a serving of muesli and top it with plant milk, berries, and banana.
6. Store the remaining muesli in a Mason jar.

Note: A handful of muesli makes a good snack.

LUNCH   MASHED CHICKPEA AND AVOCADO SANDWICH

INGREDIENTS

1   can (15 ounces) chickpeas, rinsed

1   avocado

1   small carrot, diced

Juice of 1 lemon

¼   cup hummus (optional)

1   handful of sunflower seeds

Sea salt and freshly ground pepper

Bread

Greens or sprouts

INSTRUCTIONS

1. In a medium bowl, roughly mash the chickpeas with the back of a fork.
2. Add the avocado and mash well.
3. Add the carrot, lemon juice, optional hummus, sunflower seeds, salt and pepper, and mix to combine.
4. Spread on bread.
5. Top with greens or sprouts.

Note: I always keep fresh hummus in the fridge for snacking.

DINNER   STIRRED-NOT-FRIED WILD RICE

Recipe by Darshana Thacker, courtesy of Forks Over Knives.

This vegan recipe combines wild rice and steam-fried vegetables for a healthy alternative to traditionally greasy fried rice. To make this a hearty one-dish meal, you can mix in a can of cooked black beans with the rice.

INGREDIENTS

5   ounces fresh shiitake mushrooms, stems removed and sliced

1   large white onion, cut into ½-inch pieces

2   tablespoons grated fresh ginger

1   cup uncooked wild rice, rinsed and drained

1   cup red sweet pepper, sliced into strips

¾   cup thin, bite-size carrot strips

1   clove garlic, minced

2   tablespoons reduced-sodium tamari sauce

1   tablespoon brown rice vinegar

1   cup thinly sliced napa cabbage

1   cup thinly sliced baby bok choy
¼   cup slivered green onions
¼   teaspoon freshly ground white or black pepper
1   tablespoon finely minced fresh cilantro
1   tablespoon sesame seeds

INSTRUCTIONS

1. In a medium saucepan, cook half of the mushrooms with the white onion and ginger in ¼ cup water over medium-low heat for 4 to 5 minutes or until onion is tender.
2. Add 1¾ cups water, bring to boiling, and stir in wild rice. Return to boiling, reduce heat, and simmer, covered, for 40 to 45 minutes or until rice is tender.
3. Meanwhile, in a large skillet cook peppers, carrots, and garlic in ¼ cup water for 2 to 3 minutes or until carrots are nearly tender.
4. Combine tamari sauce and vinegar. Stir into carrot mixture. Stir in cabbage, bok choy, green onions, pepper, and the remaining mushrooms. Cook 2 to 3 minutes or until cabbage and bok choy are slightly wilted.
5. Serve vegetable mixture over rice or stir it into rice. Sprinkle with cilantro and sesame seeds.

Day 12

The Plant-Based Plan: Have fruit for dessert. Frozen grapes and bananas are delicious. Mixed berries please so many. You can make frozen-banana ice cream in a high-power blender—just blend with a little liquid (plant milk, water, or juice).

BREAKFAST   EASY VEGAN CREPES

INGREDIENTS

1   flax egg (1 tablespoon ground flax mixed with 3 tablespoons water)
1   cup plant milk

1   cup all-purpose flour
Oil or oil spray
Fruit butter, nut butter, fresh fruit (for serving)

INSTRUCTIONS

1. Prepare the flax egg first so it can sit and thicken while you get the other ingredients.
2. Combine the milk and flour in a bowl. Add the flax egg. Mix well.
3. Heat a small skillet with a little oil (or spray lightly).
4. Pour a little of the batter in the pan. Tilt the skillet so the batter spreads.
5. Cook thoroughly; flip crepe over when no wet areas can be seen.
6. Cook the second side until light brown.
7. Put the crepe on a plate and repeat the process.
8. Top the crepes with fruit butter, nut butter, fresh fruit, or anything you like. Roll up and enjoy!

LUNCH   ROASTED CARROT, RED ONION, AND LENTIL SALAD

INGREDIENTS

4   carrots, peeled and sliced diagonally
2   small red onions, cut into 8 pieces
1   tablespoon olive oil
Sea salt and freshly ground pepper
⅓   cup sunflower seeds
4   ounces arugula
1   can (15 ounces) of lentils, rinsed
(or use a package from the grocery store or cook your own)
1   teaspoon ground cumin
Arugula (for serving)

CASHEW CHEESE

1 cup soaked cashews, drained (soak in water while you
  prepare the veggies)
2 tablespoons lemon juice
1 tablespoon nutritional yeast
  Sea salt and freshly ground pepper
¼ cup water

INSTRUCTIONS

1. Preheat the oven to 350 degrees.
2. Place the carrots and onions on a baking tray lined with
   parchment paper. Toss by hand with a little bit of oil, salt, and
   pepper, then roast in the oven for 30 minutes.
3. Heat a pan and toast the sunflower seeds for a few minutes on low
   until they start to brown, then set aside to cool.
4. Make the cashew cheese: Blend all the ingredients in a high-speed
   blender until totally smooth and set aside.
5. Add the lentils to the pan that held the sunflower seeds. Warm
   over gentle heat. Stir in the carrots and onion, add the cumin,
   and then season to taste with salt and pepper.
6. Remove the pan from the heat and mix in the arugula.
7. Place the salad on a plate. Sprinkle with sunflower seeds and some
   generous dollops of cashew cheese before serving.

DINNER   THREE-BEAN SALAD AND GREENS

INGREDIENTS

SALAD

1 can (15 ounces) black beans
1 can (15 ounces) garbanzo beans
1 can (15 ounces) red beans (or any combination of beans that you like)
1 red onion, chopped
2 stalks of celery, chopped
1 handful of arugula or spinach
1 bunch of parsley, chopped

DRESSING

½ cup apple cider vinegar

2 teaspoons mustard of choice

1 tablespoon maple syrup

Spices of choice, optional

INSTRUCTIONS

1. Make the dressing. Mix vinegar, mustard, and maple syrup together and adjust flavor to taste.

2. Open the cans of beans, rinse, drain, and combine.

3. Add the chopped onion and celery.

4. Add the greens of choice.

5. Combine beans, vegetables, and greens. Drizzle with dressing.

Note: You can add rice, lentils, or quinoa too.

Day 13

The Plant-Based Plan: Leftovers make great lunches. Soups and stews can be served over a baked sweet potato or white potato. You can crumble a burger and add it to a salad. A lentil loaf can be sliced and made into a sandwich; add lettuce and sprouts. Leftover vegetables can be tossed into any homemade soup or stir-fry.

BREAKFAST   GREEN SMOOTHIE 2

INGREDIENTS

1 cup plant milk (or ½ cup plant milk and ½ cup water)

¼ cup frozen berries

½ frozen banana

1 handful of spinach

1 small handful of chopped dates

Ground flax and cinnamon (optional)

INSTRUCTIONS
1. Blend all the ingredients.
2. Add more liquid if needed.

LUNCH   RAW BROCCOLI ROMAINE SALAD

INGREDIENTS

1	head broccoli, chopped (or a bag of fresh florets)
2–3	heads of romaine, chopped
½	pound of carrots, shredded
2–3	scallions, sliced
1	red pepper, seeded and chopped
¼	cup walnuts
¼	cup dried cherries

DRESSING

¼	cup sugar (or maple syrup)
¼	cup olive oil
¼	cup balsamic vinegar
2	teaspoons tamari or soy sauce

INSTRUCTIONS
1. Toss the vegetables together with the nuts and cherries.
2. Mix the dressing and pour on the salad.

DINNER   WHITE BEAN AND FENNEL "STOUP"

This is a recipe from our friend Miranda Domenguez, a strong and multi-talented young woman. A "stoup" is a cross between a soup and a stew.

INGREDIENTS

	Splash of vegetable broth
6	small potatoes, chopped in quarters
1	pint cherry tomatoes

1   fennel bulb, sliced into ¼-inch-thick slices
1   onion, thinly sliced
3   garlic cloves, minced
    Sea salt and freshly ground pepper
4   cups water (or 2 cups vegetable broth and 2 cups water)
2   teaspoon thyme
1   bay leaf
    Fresh parsley, crushed red pepper flakes (optional garnish)

INSTRUCTIONS

1. Put the broth in a stockpot. Add the potatoes, tomatoes, fennel, onion, and garlic. Season with salt and pepper. Cook on medium heat and cover with a lid. Keep covered until the tomatoes burst, about 10 to 15 minutes. Stir every few minutes.
2. Once the tomatoes have burst and the potatoes have browned, add the water, thyme, and bay leaf. Bring to a boil. Cover and simmer for 20 minutes, or until the potatoes are fork-tender.
3. When the stoup is done, remove the bay leaf. Serve and garnish with parsley and crushed red pepper, if desired.

Day 14

The Plant-Based Plan: Try different berries and spices in chia pudding and oatmeal. Rotate between cinnamon, pumpkin pie spice, and allspice.

BREAKFAST   CHIA PUDDING FOR ONE

INGREDIENTS

½   banana
½   cup berries
2   tablespoons chia seeds
½   cup plant milk
    Cinnamon, nutmeg, nuts, seeds, fruit (for serving)

INSTRUCTIONS

1. The evening before you plan to have the pudding, mash the banana and berries. (I mash them right in the small glass bowl I eat from.)
2. Add the chia and milk.
3. Mix well and add anything else you want.
4. Cover and refrigerate for the morning.
5. Before serving, top with a combination of cinnamon, nutmeg, nuts, and seeds.

Note: Cut overripe bananas into rounds. Freeze in plastic bags. You can use frozen berries and put the berries and frozen banana in a bowl to defrost in the refrigerator. Mash and mix together.

LUNCH   MINESTRONE SOUP

INGREDIENTS

1   onion, chopped

3   stalks celery, chopped

3   carrots, chopped

1   garlic clove, minced

Splash of vegetable broth

9   cups water (or water and vegetable broth)

¼   cup dry lentils, rinsed

¼   cup dry split peas, rinsed

¼   cup barley, rinsed (omit if the soup needs to be gluten-free)

1   can (8 ounces) tomato sauce

1   teaspoon balsamic vinegar

1   package (10 ounces) frozen spinach (or fresh spinach or other leafy green of choice)

2   teaspoons basil

1   teaspoon oregano

½   cup small shell pasta

INSTRUCTIONS

1. Sauté the onion, celery, carrots, and garlic in broth until tender. Set aside.
2. Heat the water to boiling in a skillet. Add the lentils, peas, and barley. Cook for 15 minutes.
3. Add the onion-garlic mixture, tomato sauce, vinegar, greens, and herbs to the soup. Cook another 15 minutes.
4. Add the pasta and cook until tender. Adjust the seasoning.

Note: Use a prepackaged mirepoix mix to save time on chopping the onion, celery, and carrots. Add a can of rinsed beans when you add the pasta. Spoon leftovers over a baked potato for another meal.

DINNER   RICE-PAPER VEGGIE ROLLS

INGREDIENTS

Carrots, spinach, cabbage, avocado, cucumber, fresh herbs (any combination)

Rice-paper wrappers

Peanut sauce and/or tahini-garlic sauce

PEANUT SAUCE

2 garlic cloves, minced
1 tablespoon fresh gingerroot, peeled and finely chopped
2 tablespoons each of tamari, maple syrup, and lime juice
   Chili powder (optional)
⅓ cup peanut butter
⅓ cup water (more or less as needed)

TAHINI-GARLIC SAUCE

2 tablespoons tahini
   Juice of 1 lime
1 garlic clove, minced
3 tablespoons water (add more if needed to desired consistency)
1 tablespoon maple syrup

INSTRUCTIONS

1. Slice the veggies in thin strips. Chop the herbs.
2. Blend ingredients for one or both sauces.
3. Dip rice-paper sheets in warm water so they soften and become pliable (do this one at a time), then arrange your fillings in the middle. Fold over two ends, then wrap the sheet up like a burrito, making it as tight as possible. It might take a few tries to get it perfect.
4. Serve with one or both sauces.

Day 15

The Plant-Based Plan: Use pizza as a decoy. The base of a pizza can be an excuse for arugula, garlic, pine nuts, sun-dried tomatoes, avocado slices, peppers, mushrooms, and eggplant. Make pizza a pizza salad.

BREAKFAST   CINNAMON ALMOND DATE BITES

Recipe by VeggieChick.com.

INGREDIENTS

½ cup oats, gluten-free if desired

2 tablespoons unsweetened cocoa

1 cup packed, pitted medjool dates (If your dates are not soft, soak them in water for 15 minutes, and then drain.)

3 tablespoons almond butter

¼ cup unsweetened coconut flakes

1 tablespoon chia seeds (or ground flax seeds)

½ teaspoon ground cinnamon

INSTRUCTIONS

1. Add oats and cocoa to food processor. Blend until coarse. Add remaining ingredients and blend until thoroughly combined.
2. Form into balls and refrigerate.
3. Store in an airtight container for up to a week.

LUNCH   SOBA NOODLE SOUP AND MUSHROOMS

INGREDIENTS

4   cups vegetable broth
4   ounces baby bella mushrooms, sliced
1   tablespoon fresh gingerroot, minced
2   garlic cloves, minced
1   teaspoon hot sauce (I like sriracha.)
3   tablespoons tamari or soy sauce
4   ounces soba noodles
3   handfuls of shredded kale or Swiss chard
    Sesame seeds

INSTRUCTIONS

1. Heat the broth over medium heat in a soup pot.
   Add the mushrooms. Cook for about 4 minutes.
2. Add the ginger, garlic, and hot sauce to the soup pot.
   Cook for another minute.
3. Add the tamari and stir so nothing sticks to the pot.
   Cook another few minutes.
4. Bring to a boil and reduce to a simmer. Add the noodles
   and the greens. Cook for about 5 minutes, or until the noodles
   are tender.
5. Remove from the heat. Spoon into bowls. Sprinkle sesame seeds
   on top.

Note: Top the soup with leftover cooked quinoa.

DINNER   QUINOA PIZZA

INGREDIENTS

CRUST

¾	cup quinoa
½	teaspoon sea salt
½	teaspoon freshly ground pepper
1	garlic clove
2	teaspoons oregano
¼	cup water
¼	cup vegan cheese, shredded
1	tablespoon olive oil
	Marinara sauce (enough to cover the crust)
	Pizza toppings of your choice

INSTRUCTIONS

1. Put the quinoa in a fine-mesh strainer. Place the strainer in a bowl. Fill the bowl with water to cover the quinoa. Let it soak overnight.
2. The next day, preheat the oven to 375 degrees.
3. Line a baking sheet with parchment paper.
4. Drain and rinse the quinoa. Put the quinoa in a blender with salt, pepper, garlic, oregano, and water. Blend. It should be the consistency of pancake batter.
5. Pour the batter into a bowl. Add the cheese and olive oil and stir well.
6. Line a round tart pan with parchment paper, and pour the batter onto the parchment, with the ring of the pan to define the pizza.
7. Bake for 20 minutes. Remove the crust from the oven and flip it into a second pan, also lined with parchment, to cook the other side.
8. Bake crust another 5 to 10 minutes. Remove it from the oven.
9. Lower the oven temperature to 345 degrees.
10. Add the marinara sauce and toppings to the crust and bake for another 5 to 8 minutes.

Day 16

The Plant-Based Plan: Keep bags of frozen broccoli and cauliflower stocked to always have members of the cruciferous family handy. Add them to soups, casseroles, stir-fries, and pizza toppings. This is one of the healthiest families of foods.

BREAKFAST   OATMEAL BAKE

This makes a full baking dish. I cut it up into squares and take one or two for breakfast.

INGREDIENTS

- 2 cups rolled oats
- 2 cups plant milk
- 4 tablespoons chia seeds
- 2 teaspoons cinnamon
- 1 large apple, chopped or grated
- 3 tablespoons dried cherries or raisins
- 1 teaspoon vanilla extract
- 1–2 teaspoons maple syrup

INSTRUCTIONS

1. Preheat the oven to 400 degrees.
2. Mix all the ingredients together. Stir well to mix the chia seeds evenly. Pour into a 9-by-9-inch lightly oiled baking dish.
3. Bake covered for 20 minutes. Uncover and cook another 20 minutes.
4. Let cool and cut into squares.

Note: You can switch up the fruit and spices. Try pears, for example, and use pumpkin pie spice and cranberries.

LUNCH   EASY LENTIL SOUP

This is so easy and delicious. It is even better the second day.

INGREDIENTS

 1   prepackaged mirepoix mix (16 ounces)
      (or 2 carrots, 3 celery stalks, and 1 onion, all chopped)
 3   quarts vegetable broth
1½ cups dry red lentils
      Pinch of thyme
 1   teaspoon ground cumin
      Sea salt and freshly ground pepper

INSTRUCTIONS

1. In a soup pot, sauté the mirepoix in a little of the broth for a few minutes.
2. Rinse the lentils and add them to the pot with the remaining broth.
3. Add the seasonings. Cover and simmer about 30 minutes.

Note: Throw in a handful a spinach just before the soup is done cooking.

DINNER   POTATO AND CAULIFLOWER CURRY (ALOO GOBI)

INGREDIENTS

 1   onion, diced
 1   teaspoon turmeric
 1   ½-inch slice fresh gingerroot, grated
      Splash of vegetable broth
 1   tablespoon curry powder
 3   garlic cloves, minced
 1   teaspoon ground cumin
 1   teaspoon ground coriander
 3   medium potatoes, cut into bite-size pieces

½   cauliflower head, broken into florets

1   can (15 ounces) tomato purée (or 3 fresh tomatoes)

¾   cup frozen peas

INSTRUCTIONS

1. Sauté the onion, turmeric, and ginger in the broth on medium heat. Cover and cook for a few minutes.

2. Add the curry powder, garlic, cumin, and coriander and continue cooking on low heat for about 2–3 minutes.

3. Add the potatoes and cauliflower and stir. Cover and cook on low heat for about 5 minutes.

4. Add the tomato purée, and continue to cook on low for about 15 minutes, or until the vegetables are soft.

5. Stir in the peas. Mix gently. Cook covered for another few minutes.

Day 17

The Plant-Based Plan: Grate your veggies. Add grated carrots, parsnips, or squash to the preparation of any dish (this works especially well with lasagna, veggie loaves, burrito fillings, and of course salads) to add the fiber and nutrients found only in plants. Be brave and try grated beets (perfect for veggie burgers)!

BREAKFAST   CHIA BRAN MUFFINS

This recipe was created by our wonderful friend Monni, photographer extraordinaire and dog lover. She makes these every week, and they freeze well.

INGREDIENTS

4–5   ripe bananas (mashed)

10   ounces nondairy vanilla yogurt (Monni uses Silk brand vanilla soy yogurt.)

⅓   cup canola oil

  1   cup unsweetened applesauce
  5   ounces agave syrup (or maple syrup)
  ¾ teaspoon sea salt
  1   cup all-purpose flour
  1   cup 100 percent whole-wheat flour
  ¾ cup wheat-bran flakes
  1   tablespoon baking powder
1⅔ cups chia seeds
      Approximately 2 cups raspberries or blueberries
      or a combination of both

INSTRUCTIONS

1. Preheat the oven to 350 degrees.
2. Line a muffin pan with liners for 12 to 15 muffins.
3. In one bowl mash the bananas, then add yogurt, oil, applesauce, and agave, and mix it all together.
4. In a separate bowl, mix the salt, flours, bran flakes, baking powder, and chia seeds.
5. Mix the wet mixture into the dry mixture and get the lumps out. Stir in the fruit carefully so as not to smash it.
6. Let the mixture sit for at least 20 minutes.
7. Scoop the muffin mixture into the muffin liners.
8. Bake for 1 hour, or until a toothpick comes out clean. Take the muffins out of the oven and allow to cool.

LUNCH   SPICY BAKED POTATO WITH BROCCOLI AND VEGAN QUESO

Recipe by VeggieChick.com.

INGREDIENTS

  2   medium russet potatoes
  8   ounces broccolini
      Jalapeño hot sauce, to taste

VEGAN QUESO

1½	cups raw cashews
3	tablespoons nutritional yeast
¼	cup fresh lemon juice
1	can (15 ounces) great northern beans (or pinto beans), rinsed and drained
1	tablespoon tahini (optional)
2	teaspoons jalapeño hot sauce
1	teaspoon turmeric
1	teaspoon onion powder
½	teaspoon garlic powder
½	teaspoon Spanish paprika
¼	teaspoon sea salt
¾–1	cup hot water

INSTRUCTIONS

1. Cook potatoes as desired (microwave, bake, boil, Instant Pot, etc.).
2. Steam the broccolini until just starting to get soft.
3. Prepare the queso. Add cashews to a food processor and process on high for 2 to 3 minutes, stopping to scrape the sides as necessary. The cashews will start to resemble a butterlike consistency. Add the nutritional yeast, lemon juice, beans, tahini, hot sauce, spices, and hot water. Blend again until smooth. If still not smooth, add more water in 1-tablespoon increments and blend.
4. To prepare baked potatoes, cut a slit in each potato lengthwise and break away the skin to expose the flesh. Press with a fork. Add the broccoli and drizzle the queso on top. If desired, top with jalapeño hot sauce or additional spices.

Note: This recipe makes about 2 cups of queso.

DINNER HEARTY CHILI

INGREDIENTS

- 1   carrot, peeled and chopped
- 1   medium yellow onion, diced
- ½   cup vegetable broth for sautéing
- 3   cloves garlic, minced
- ½   cup bulgur, rinsed (or lentils if you want this dish to be gluten-free, but the bulgur gives thick, delicious consistency)
- ½–1   cup water (plus more if needed)
- 1   sweet potato, peeled, cut into bite-size pieces
- 2   tablespoons chili powder
- 1   tablespoon ground cumin
- 1   tablespoon brown sugar
- ¼   teaspoon cayenne powder
- 2   cans (28 ounces) diced tomatoes (I use Pomi brand or Thrive Market brand.)
- 1   can (15 ounces) tomato sauce (I use Pomi brand, which comes in a box.)
- 1   can (15 ounces) black beans, drained and rinsed (I use Eden Organic brand.)
- 1   can (15 ounces) kidney beans, drained and rinsed

INSTRUCTIONS

1. Sauté the onion and carrots in broth in a medium-size pot, stirring often, until the onion is soft and translucent, about 5 minutes.
2. Add the garlic and sauté for 1 minute. Add the bulgur, water, sweet potato, chili powder, cumin, brown sugar, and cayenne. Stir until well combined. (If you use lentils instead of bulgur, you probably will not need to add the water.)
3. Add the tomatoes, tomato sauce, and beans. Bring to a boil, then reduce the heat, cover, and simmer, stirring occasionally, until the sweet potato can be pierced with a fork, about 45 minutes.
4. Season to taste.

Day 18

The Plant-Based Plan: Freeze some grapes. Grapes contain the chemical resveratrol, which is usually credited for the positive health effects of red wine and may slow aging and improve heart health. This is especially true for red grapes. Frozen grapes make a delicious snack that is sweet, cold, and quite pleasing. You can even add them to a cold glass of water or wine to act as a plant ice cube.

BREAKFAST AVOCADO TOAST

INGREDIENTS

2 slices of your favorite bread (We use Ezekiel brand.)
1 avocado
   Sea salt and freshly ground pepper
   Hemp seeds and red chili flakes (optional)

INSTRUCTIONS

1. Toast the bread.
2. Mash the avocado. Season to taste.
3. Spread on the warm toast.
4. Sprinkle with hemp seeds and chili flakes.

LUNCH CAULIFLOWER STIR-FRY

INGREDIENTS

1 head of cauliflower, cut into florets
1 tablespoon olive oil or canola oil
   Sea salt and freshly ground pepper
2 tablespoons vegetable broth
4–6 small pieces of fresh gingerroot
3 garlic cloves, minced
1 small onion, chopped
2 scallions, cut into 1- to 2-inch pieces
½ teaspoon red pepper flakes

 1 teaspoon toasted sesame oil
 2 tablespoons rice wine
1½ tablespoons tamari or soy sauce
 ¼ teaspoon sugar
    Steamed rice (for serving)

INSTRUCTIONS

1. Preheat the oven to 450 degrees.
2. Line a baking tray with parchment paper.
3. Place the cauliflower in a single layer on the parchment. Toss gently with the oil. Season with salt and pepper and roast for about 25 minutes.
4. Heat a wok with the broth. Add the ginger. After a few minutes add the garlic and onion. Stir so they do not burn.
5. Turn the heat up and add the roasted cauliflower and scallions. Add the pepper flakes, sesame oil, wine, tamari, and sugar.
6. Stir everything for about 1 minute.
7. Serve with steamed rice.

Note: You can also throw in spinach or leftover broccoli toward the end of the cooking.

DINNER   NACHOS

INGREDIENTS
CHIPS

Corn tortillas, cut into triangles
Juice of 1 lime
Salt
Chili powder
Ground cumin

NACHO "CHEESE" SAUCE

 1 small red pepper, deseeded and chopped
 1 teaspoon chili powder
 ½ teaspoon cayenne
 ½ teaspoon sea salt
    Juice of ½ lemon
 4 tablespoons nutritional yeast
 4 tablespoons hemp seeds
 1 garlic clove, minced
 ⅓ cup water

NACHOS

    Chips
    Nacho "cheese" sauce
    Fresh pico de gallo, salsa, or chopped tomato
    Black beans or pinto beans, rinsed
    Chopped cilantro
    Hot sauce
    Sliced avocado or guacamole (optional)

INSTRUCTIONS
 1. Preheat the oven to 450 degrees.
 2. Place the cut tortillas on a pan. Sprinkle with lime juice
    and spices.
 3. Bake for 5 to 7 minutes, or until they start to crisp.
 4. Make the cheese sauce: Blend all the ingredients in a high-speed
    blender until smooth. You want to use just enough water to get
    the mixture smooth. Blend 30 to 40 seconds and taste. If it's
    still grainy, blend with a bit more water. Place the sauce in the
    refrigerator for a few hours, or until it thickens (best to make
    the day before).
 5. Lay out the nacho chips on a plate and pile all the nacho
    ingredients on top.

Day 19

The Plant-Based Plan: Need a fast meal? Take a steamed collard green or a 100 percent whole-wheat tortilla and pack it with hummus, vegetables, and salsa (or the tabouli below). I even add mustard. Kids love the collards, and they hold up well as a wrapper for sandwiches.

BREAKFAST BREAKFAST BLUEBERRY-QUINOA FLAKES

INGREDIENTS

⅓ cup quinoa flakes (We use Ancient Harvest brand, which is available at most grocery stores.)

1 cup water

½ cup frozen blueberries

Pinch of cinnamon

INSTRUCTIONS

1. Put all the ingredients in a small saucepan.
2. Bring to a boil and reduce the heat to simmer. This will cook in about 1 minute!

LUNCH CHICKPEA AND QUINOA TABOULI

INGREDIENTS

1 pint cherry tomatoes

1 cup fresh parsley, chopped

1 cup spinach, chopped

½ red onion, chopped

1 large cucumber, chopped

1 can (15 ounces) chickpeas, rinsed

½ cup cooked quinoa

DRESSING
- 2 tablespoons olive oil
- Juice of 3 lemons
- ½ teaspoon garlic, minced
- ½ teaspoon sea salt
- ¼ teaspoon freshly ground pepper

INSTRUCTIONS
1. Chop the tomatoes into small pieces.
2. Mix the tomatoes with the parsley, spinach, onion, cucumber, and chickpeas.
3. Stir in the quinoa and dressing.

DINNER   MAC AND "CHEESE"

INGREDIENTS
- 1 box (1 pound) of your favorite pasta
- 1 cup spinach
- Other veggies (optional)
- Cheese sauce (recipe below)

CHEESE SAUCE
- 1 tablespoon buttery spread (We use Earth Balance brand.)
- 1 tablespoon flour (You can use gluten-free flour.)
- 1 cup room-temperature plant milk
- ½ teaspoon turmeric
- ½ teaspoon paprika
- Sea salt and freshly ground pepper
- 4 ounces vegan cheese, shredded (We use Daiya brand.)

INSTRUCTIONS
1. Cook the pasta per box instructions.
2. Remove the pasta from the heat and drain. Add the spinach and optional other veggies to the pot of pasta. Cover while you make the cheese sauce.

3. Make the cheese sauce: Melt the spread in a pot over low heat. Whisk in the flour. Add the milk and spices. Stir and cook until it thickens. Add salt and pepper. Add the cheese and stir till it melts.
4. Pour the sauce over the pasta and serve.

Day 20

The Plant-Based Plan: Keep a few bags of frozen organic greens in your freezer. Frozen greens are inexpensive, won't spoil, and often do not have to be washed. They can be used in soups, pasta sauces, and burrito fillings.

BREAKFAST BLUEBERRY-BUCKWHEAT BREAKFAST

Buckwheat groats are the hulled, gluten-free seeds from the buckwheat plant, which is related to rhubarb. The robust flavor of this quick-cooking, gluten-free grain is perfect for salads, soups, and cereal.

INGREDIENTS
1 cup buckwheat groats, soaked overnight
2 cups blueberries
2 tablespoons maple syrup
½ cup almond milk or water
1 banana
Juice of ½ lemon
1 teaspoon vanilla
Berries or seeds

INSTRUCTIONS
1. Drain buckwheat groats and rinse well.
2. Blend the blueberries with the maple syrup until very smooth. Remove about ¼ cup of the blueberry purée and set aside.

3. Add the buckwheat groats, milk, banana, lemon juice, and vanilla to the remaining blueberry purée in the blender and blend until smooth.
4. Pour the buckwheat mixture into bowls and swirl in the remaining purée.
5. Top with berries or seeds.

LUNCH SOBA NOODLE AND RAW VEGGIE SALAD

INGREDIENTS

8	ounces soba noodles
3–4	scallions, sliced
¾	cup chopped cilantro
1	red bell pepper, thinly sliced
¼	head of red cabbage, thinly sliced
3	whole carrots, shredded with vegetable peeler
2	cups shelled edamame, steamed
½	cup tamari or soy sauce
2	teaspoons sesame oil
2	tablespoons rice wine vinegar
	Juice of 1 lime
1½	teaspoons red pepper flakes
½	cup toasted sesame seeds

INSTRUCTIONS

1. Cook the soba noodles according to package instructions. Drain and rinse.
2. Chop all the veggies. Combine the veggies and soba noodles in a bowl.
3. Whisk together the tamari, sesame oil, rice wine vinegar, pepper flakes, and lime juice.
4. Toast the sesame seeds in the toaster oven. Watch carefully because they burn quickly.
5. Pour the dressing on the salad, and top with the toasted sesame seeds.

DINNER   TASTY PAELLA

INGREDIENTS

½ teaspoon saffron threads (I get them at Trader Joe's.)

3 tablespoons warm water

2½ cups vegetable broth, divided

1 medium onion, sliced

1 yellow bell pepper, sliced

1 red bell pepper, sliced

1 cup mushrooms, sliced

3 cloves garlic, minced

Sea salt and freshly ground pepper, to taste

1 cup short-grain rice

2 Roma tomatoes, chopped, or 1 can or box (14 ounces) diced tomatoes

1½ teaspoons smoked paprika

½ cup green peas (fresh or defrosted)

1 can (15 ounces) artichoke hearts in water, drained and chopped

1 can (15 ounces) garbanzo beans, rinsed and drained (I use Eden Organic brand.)

½ cup parsley, chopped

INSTRUCTIONS

1. In a small bowl, combine the saffron and water. Let steep for 10 minutes.

2. In a medium saucepan, heat a splash of broth. Add the onion and sauté for 2 minutes. Add peppers and continue to sauté until soft, about 5 minutes. Add the mushrooms and garlic and sauté for 5 minutes or until the mushrooms soften and release liquid. Season with salt and pepper.

3. Increase heat to medium-high. Add one-third of the broth. Then add the rice, tomatoes, and smoked paprika.

4. Reduce heat to medium-low. Stir in the saffron water. Simmer uncovered for 5 minutes or until the broth is almost completely absorbed.

5. Add another third of the broth and simmer uncovered for 5 minutes or until the liquid is almost completely absorbed.

6. Add the remaining third of broth and cook for 5 to 10 minutes.

7. Add the garbanzo beans and stir to combine. Sprinkle peas and artichoke hearts over top.

8. Cover the pan tightly with foil and cook over low heat for 12 minutes.

9. Turn the heat off, leave the foil in place, and let the paella rest for 10 minutes.

10. Remove the foil and top with parsley.

Note: You can add leftover spinach or any other veggies when you add the peas.

Day 21

The Plant-Based Plan: Try grilled fruit for dessert. While grilled meat is known to be unhealthy, grilled pineapple, peaches, bananas, and even apples hold up well and open a new door to more servings of plants.

BREAKFAST   PUMPKIN PIE BREAKFAST QUINOA

INGREDIENTS

⅓   cup quinoa flakes

⅓   cup pumpkin purée

1   tablespoon maple syrup

1¼   cups plant milk or water

½   teaspoon vanilla extract

1   teaspoon pumpkin pie spice

INSTRUCTIONS

1. Mix the quinoa flakes, pumpkin, maple syrup, and milk in a saucepan, and bring to boil.
2. Reduce heat and simmer. Add the vanilla. This cooks quickly, so don't walk away from the stove.
3. Stir and then remove from the heat. Add the spice.

LUNCH   APPLE SLAW

INGREDIENTS

1	cup shredded cabbage
1	medium carrot, shredded
1	apple, shredded
¼	red onion, chopped
2	tablespoons raisins
2	tablespoons pumpkin seeds
2	tablespoons tahini
2	tablespoons tamari or soy sauce
1	teaspoon mustard
	Sea salt and freshly ground pepper
	Parsley (garnish)

INSTRUCTIONS

1. Combine all the ingredients together.
2. Garnish with parsley.

DINNER   POPCORN CAULIFLOWER

This recipe is from the awesome Jill Greenbaum, sister extraordinaire.

INGREDIENTS

2   heads of cauliflower, chopped into florets

2   tablespoons extra-virgin olive oil or organic canola oil (optional)

SEASONING

1   teaspoon sea salt

2   teaspoons sugar

¼   teaspoon onion powder

¼   teaspoon garlic powder

½   teaspoon paprika

½   teaspoon turmeric

INSTRUCTIONS

1. Preheat the oven to 400 degrees.
2. Mix the seasoning spices together and set aside.
3. Place cauliflower florets on parchment paper.
4. Drizzle the cauliflower with oil if desired. Toss gently.
5. Sprinkle with the seasoning.
6. Bake for 30 to 35 minutes.

Note: I make a large batch of the spice mix and fill an empty spice jar with it. You can use it to roast other vegetables, such as potatoes, sweet potatoes, carrots, and broccoli.

Bonus Recipes

TEX-MEX SPAGHETTI SQUASH WITH BLACK BEAN GUACAMOLE

From drjoelkahn.com.

INGREDIENTS

- 1 medium spaghetti squash
- Vegetable broth
- Sea salt and freshly ground pepper

BLACK BEAN GUACAMOLE

- 2 avocados, flesh scooped out
- ½ cup red onion, chopped
- 1 small tomato, seeded and chopped
- 1 can (15 ounces) black beans, rinsed
- ¼ cup chopped cilantro
- 2 tablespoons fresh lime juice, or to taste
- Sea salt and freshly ground pepper
- Red pepper flakes
- Chili powder
- Ground cumin
- Oregano

INSTRUCTIONS

1. Preheat the oven to 375 degrees.
2. Line a large baking sheet with parchment paper.
3. Slice off the stem of the squash and place the squash cut side down on a cutting board. With a chef's knife, carefully slice through the squash lengthwise to create two long halves. Scoop out the seeds. Brush some vegetable broth onto the squash and sprinkle with salt and pepper.
4. Place squash halves cut side down on the baking sheet and roast for 30 to 50 minutes, depending on how large your squash is.

When the squash is tender and you can easily scrape the strands with a fork, it's ready. Be sure not to cook too long or it will turn mushy.

5. While the squash is roasting, prepare the black bean guacamole: Mash the avocado in a large bowl. Fold in the onion, tomato, beans, and cilantro. Season to taste with lime juice, salt, pepper, and red pepper flakes.

6. Remove the squash from the oven, flip over, and scrape the flesh with a fork in vertical motions. Do this until you've scraped all the strands off the skin. Sprinkle with chili powder, cumin, oregano, salt, and pepper (as much or as little as you want). Top the squash with guacamole and serve warm.

SMOKY BUTTERNUT SQUASH SAUCE WITH PASTA AND GREENS

From drjoelkahn.com.

INGREDIENTS

1   butternut squash (3½ to 4 pounds), peeled, seeded, and diced (or 2 packages, 10 ounces each, chopped fresh squash)

¼   cup raw cashews, soaked 3 to 4 hours or overnight, drained

¾   cup water

2   garlic cloves

2   tablespoons nutritional yeast (optional, but recommended)

1   tablespoon lemon juice

½   teaspoon onion powder

½   teaspoon smoked paprika

¼   teaspoon chili powder

⅛   teaspoon liquid smoke

Hot sauce

1   package (10 ounces) 100 percent whole-grain mini shells or macaroni pasta

Roasted broccoli or sautéed kale leaves

INSTRUCTIONS

1. Preheat the oven to 425 degrees.
2. Line a baking sheet with parchment paper.
3. Spread the chopped squash on the sheet. Roast for 30 to 40 minutes, flipping once halfway through baking, until the squash is fork-tender. Let cool for at least 5 minutes.
4. Put the cashews, water, garlic, optional nutritional yeast, lemon juice, onion powder, paprika, chili powder, and 2 cups of the cooked squash into a high-speed blender. Blend on high until smooth. Add the liquid smoke and hot sauce to taste and blend again.
5. Cook the pasta according to package directions.
6. Add the drained pasta back into the pot. Pour the desired amount of sauce on the pasta and stir to combine. Stir in the broccoli or kale. Cook over medium until heated through and serve immediately.

THE WORLD'S BEST OIL-FREE BABA GANOUSH

From GreenSpace Café, Ferndale, Michigan.

INGREDIENTS

2–3 medium eggplants (about 3 pounds total)
⅓ cup tahini (optional)
2 garlic cloves
Juice of 2 lemons (about ½ cup)
Sea salt and freshly ground pepper

INSTRUCTIONS

1. Preheat the oven to 450 degrees.
2. Place the eggplants in a roasting pan and pierce them with a fork. Roast the eggplants until the skin has charred and the interior is tender, 15 to 20 minutes. Let cool.

3. Peel and seed the cooled eggplant, roughly chop the flesh, and then transfer it to the bowl of a food processor.

4. Into the processor bowl add the tahini, garlic, lemon juice, salt and pepper to taste, and a few teaspoons of cold water. Process the mixture to a coarse paste, adding a bit more water as needed to allow the mixture to blend.

5. Adjust the seasoning with salt and pepper to taste and serve with crackers, vegetable slices, or on a salad.

GREENSPACE SUPERFOOD SALAD

From GreenSpace Café, Ferndale, Michigan.

INGREDIENTS

6 ounces baby kale

½ sweet potato, roasted

2 florets of broccolini, roasted

1 cup cooked quinoa

Few pinches of any kind of fresh sprouts

¼ avocado, sliced

1 tablespoon hemp seeds

¼ cup walnuts, toasted

BALSAMIC DRESSING

From Jane Esselstyn.

3 tablespoons balsamic vinegar

2 tablespoons Dijon mustard

1 tablespoon maple syrup

INSTRUCTIONS

1. Arrange the salad ingredients in a serving dish.

2. Mix dressing ingredients vigorously in a jar.

3. Toss the salad and dressing together, or serve dressing on the side.

WHITE BEAN OIL-FREE BASIL PESTO

From GreenSpace Café, Ferndale, Michigan.

INGREDIENTS
- 2 cups cooked white beans
- 3 cups chopped fresh basil
- Sea salt and freshly ground pepper
- Squeeze of lemon
- 1 tablespoon nutritional yeast
- Vegetable slices or seed crackers (for serving)

INSTRUCTIONS
1. Mix all the ingredients together in a bowl with a fork, making the beans creamy.
2. Serve on vegetable slices or with crackers.

Time to Grow Your
Plant-Based Health

We are at the end of a journey, but my hope is that you are at a beginning. Maybe you have been mostly or completely plant-based but had not thought much about the environment or the way animals are treated in CAFOs, whether for food production or leather. Maybe you were aware of the nauseating videos of animals tortured to make shearling winter boots and coats but did not appreciate the wealth of data supporting the potential for superior health with WFPB diets. Maybe you really are just sick and tired of being sick and tired, taking many prescription drugs a day, and are looking for a scientifically supported lifestyle that is not just a detox for seven days but for a lifetime.

Whatever the reason you picked up this book, it is my hope that you are committed to choosing plants over animals. You now know more than what most health providers know about the powerful steps to maintain or regain your health without depending on medicines, hospitalizations, or procedures. (If you are looking for a plant-based health provider, there are helpful websites like plantbaseddocs.com.) You have the mojo, the magic, the formula, and the path to live your life to the fullest and enjoy the best odds of a long lifespan and healthspan. The Plant-Based Solution is a gift to your body and soul, and it is a gift to give with kindness to others. It will always be more powerful when combined with yoga, exercise, sound sleep, and mindfulness. Wishing you health, peace, and meaning that begins on the plate, fork, and spoon.

Acknowledgments

Many people have contributed in one fashion or another to this book, whether knowingly or not. None has been of more assistance than my wife of over three decades, Karen. Her careful reading and preparation of the recipes and eating plan reflects her experience as a health teacher and head of kitchen in the Kahn household. I have been fortunate to have amazing mentors, many mentioned here, like Drs. Neal Barnard, John McDougall, Dean Ornish, Caldwell Esselstyn, and David Katz. Paul Chatlin met with me a few years back and founded the largest plant-based support group in the world, the Plant Based Nutrition Support Group, found at pbnsg.org. My son Daniel has brought GreenSpace Café from idea to reality. My children Jacob, Jessica, and Yany provide the reason to search for healthy ways to live free of chronic disease. Jake and Eva, rescue dogs, remind me of the love of animals and the need to treat them all with respect. My mother, Ruth, is an inspiration to so many and was an early adopter of healthy food for healing. Her support has been bountiful, and I send much love to her. My nurse, Jennifer Dowd, RN, BSN, MSN, provides superior care to so many at the Kahn Center for Cardiac Longevity.

Notes

Chapter 1: The Six Pillars of Support for the Plant-Based Solution

1. US Department of Health and Human Services and US Department of Agriculture, *2015–2020 Dietary Guidelines for Americans*, 8th ed, December 2015, health.gov/dietaryguidelines/2015/.

2. V. Melina, W. Craig, and S. Levin, "Position of the Academy of Nutrition and Dietetics: Vegetarian Diets," *Journal of the Academy of Nutrition and Dietetics* 116, no. 12 (December 2016): 1970–80, doi: 10.1016/j.jand.2016.09.025.

3. Ibid.

4. "Intensive Cardiac Rehabilitation (ICR) Programs," Centers for Medicare & Medicaid Services, last modified August 18, 2015, cms.gov/Medicare/Medicare -General-Information/MedicareApprovedFacilitie/ICR.html.

5. "*U.S. News & World Report* Reveals the 2016 Best Diets Rankings," *U.S. News & World Report*, January 5, 2016, usnews.com/info/blogs/press-room/2016/01/05 /us-news-reveals-the-2016-best-diets-rankings.

6. "Ornish Diet," *U.S. News & World Report*, accessed 5/22/17, health.usnews .com/best-diet/ornish-diet.

7. Phillip J. Tuso et al., "Nutritional Update for Physicians: Plant-Based Diets," *The Permanente Journal* 17, no. 2 (Spring 2013): 61–66, doi: 10.7812/TPP/12-085; Kaiser Permanente, *The Plant-Based Diet Booklet*, accessed 5/22/17, share.kaiserpermanente.org/wp-content /uploads/2015/10/The-Plant-Based-Diet-booklet.pdf.

8. Dagfinn Aune et al., "Fruit and Vegetable Intake and the Risk of Cardiovascular Disease, Total Cancer and All-Cause Mortality—A Systematic Review and Dose-Response Meta-Analysis of Prospective Studies," *International Journal of Epidemiology* (2017): 1–28, doi: 10.1093/ije/dyw319.

Chapter 2: The Heart of the Matter

1. W. Kempner et al., "Treatment of Massive Obesity with Rice/Reduction Diet Program: An Analysis of 106 Patients with at Least a 45-kg Weight Loss," *Archives of Internal Medicine* 135, no. 12 (December 1975): 1575–84, doi:10.1001/archinte.1975.00330120053008.

2. L. M. Morrison, "Reduction of Mortality Rate in Coronary Atherosclerosis by a Low Cholesterol–Low Fat Diet," *American Heart Journal* 42, no. 4 (October 1951): 538–45, doi: dx.doi.org/10.1016/0002-8703(51)90150-0.

3. R. J. Barnard et al., "Long-Term Use of a High-Complex-Carbohydrate, High-Fiber, Low-Fat Diet and Exercise in the Treatment of NIDDM Patients," *Diabetes Care* 6, no. 3 (May–June 1983): 268–73, ncbi.nlm.nih.gov/pubmed/6307614.

4. D. Ornish et al., "Effects of Stress Management Training and Dietary Changes in Treating Ischemic Heart Disease," *Journal of the American Medical Association* 249, no. 1 (January 1983): 54–59, doi:10.1001/jama.1983.03330250034024.

5. D. Ornish et al., "Can Lifestyle Changes Reverse Coronary Heart Disease? The Lifestyle Heart Trial," *The Lancet* 336, no. 8708 (July 1990): 129–33, doi: dx.doi.org/10.1016/0140-6736(90)91656-U.

6. D. Ornish et al., "Intensive Lifestyle Changes for Reversal of Coronary Heart Disease," *Journal of the American Medical Association* 280, no. 23 (December 1998): 2001–07, doi:10.1001/jama.280.23.2001.

7. Ibid.

8. C. B. Esselstyn, Jr., et al., "A Way to Reverse CAD?" *The Journal of Family Practice* 63, no. 7 (July 2014): 356–64b, ncbi.nlm.nih.gov/pubmed/25198208.

9. "Saturated Fats," American Heart Association, last updated March 24, 2017, healthyforgood.heart.org/Eat-smart/Articles/Saturated-Fats.

10. Ibid.

11. J. T. Sutliffe et al., "Nutrient-Dense, Plant-Rich Dietary Intervention Effective at Reducing Cardiovascular Disease Risk Factors for Worksites: A Pilot Study," *Alternative Therapies in Health and Medicine* 22, no. 5 (September 2016): 32–36, ncbi.nlm.nih.gov/pubmed/27622958.

12. R. A. Vogel, M. C. Corretti, and G. D. Plotnick, "Effect of a Single High -Fat Meal on Endothelial Function in Healthy Subjects," *American Journal of Cardiology* 79, no. 3 (February 1997): 350–54, doi: 10.1016 /S0002-9149(96)00760-6.

13. C. E. Cho et al., "Trimethylamine-N-oxide (TMAO) Response to Animal Source Foods Varies Among Healthy Young Men and Is Influenced by Their Gut Microbiota Composition: A Randomized Controlled Trial," *Molecular Nutrition & Food Research* 61, no. 1 (January 2017), doi: 10.1002/mnfr.201600324.

Chapter 3: The Sweet News about Diabetes

1. "More than 29 Million Americans Have Diabetes; 1 in 4 Doesn't Know It," Centers for Disease Control and Prevention, June 10, 2014, cdc.gov/media/releases/2014/p0610-diabetes-report.html.

2. "Prediabetes: Could It Be You?" Centers for Disease Control and Prevention, cdc.gov/diabetes/pubs/statsreport14/prediabetes-infographic.pdf.

3. Joseph L. Dieleman et al., "US Spending on Personal Health Care and Public Health, 1996–2013," *Journal of the American Medical Association* 316, no. 24 (December 2016): 2627–46, doi:10.1001/jama.2016.16885.

4. J. Shirley Sweeney, "Dietary Factors That Influence the Dextrose Tolerance Test: A Preliminary Study," *Archives of Internal Medicine* 40, no. 6 (1927): 818–30, doi:10.1001/archinte.1927.00130120077005.

5. Gerald I. Shulman, "Ectopic Fat in Insulin Resistance, Dyslipidemia, and Cardiometabolic Disease,"*New England Journal of Medicine* 371 (2014): 1131–41, doi: 10.1056/NEJMra1011035.

6. N. D. Barnard et al., "A Low-Fat Vegan Diet Improves Glycemic Control and Cardiovascular Risk Factors in a Randomized Clinical Trial in Individuals with Type 2 Diabetes," *Diabetes Care* 29, no 8 (August 2006): 1777–83, doi: 10.2337/dc06-0606.

7. D. A. Snowdon and R. L. Phillips, "Does a Vegetarian Diet Reduce the Occurrence of Diabetes?" *American Journal of Public Health* 75, no. 5 (May 1985): 507–12, doi: 10.2105/AJPH.75.5.507.

8. A. Vang et al., "Meats, Processed Meats, Obesity, Weight Gain and Occurrence of Diabetes Among Adults: Findings from Adventist Health Studies," *Annals of Nutrition and Metabolism* 52, no. 2 (March 2008): 96–104, doi: 10.1159/000121365.

9. S. Tonstad et al., "Type of Vegetarian Diet, Body Weight, and Prevalence of Type 2 Diabetes," *Diabetes Care* 32, no. 5 (May 2009): 791–96, doi: 10.2337/dc08-1886.

10. A. Pan et al., "Red Meat Consumption and Risk of Type 2 Diabetes: 3 Cohorts of US Adults and an Updated Meta-Analysis," *American Journal of Clinical Nutrition* 94, no. 4 (October 2011): 1088–96, doi: 10.3945/ajcn.111.018978.

11. M. B. Schulze et al., "Processed Meat and Incidence of Type 2 Diabetes in Younger and Middle-Aged Women," *Diabetologia* 46, no. 11 (November 2003): 1465–73, doi: 10.1007/s00125-003-1220-7.

12. Ibid.

13. M. Kaushik et al., "Long-Chain Omega-3 Fatty Acids, Fish Intake, and the Risk of Type 2 Diabetes Mellitus," *American Journal of Clinical Nutrition* 90, no. 3 (September 2009): 613–20, doi: 10.3945/ajcn.2008.27424.

14. S. H. Ley et al., "Associations Between Red Meat Intake and Biomarkers of Inflammation and Glucose Metabolism in Women," *American Journal of Clinical Nutrition* 99, no. 2 (February 2014): 352–60, doi: 10.3945/ajcn.113.075663.

15. S. H. Holt, J. C. Miller, and P. Petocz, "An Insulin Index of Foods: The Insulin Demand Generated by 1000-kJ Portions of Common Foods," *American Journal of Clinical Nutrition* 66, no. 5 (November 1997): 1264 –76, ncbi.nlm.nih.gov/pubmed/9356547.

16. N. E. Allen et al., "The Associations of Diet with Serum Insulin-Like Growth Factor I and Its Main Binding Proteins in 292 Women Meat-Eaters, Vegetarians, and Vegans," *Cancer Epidemiology, Biomarkers & Prevention* 11, no. 11 (November 2002): 1441–48, ncbi.nlm.nih.gov/pubmed/12433724.

17. M. F. McCarty, J. Barroso-Aranda, and F. Contreras, "The Low-Methionine Content of Vegan Diets May Make Methionine Restriction Feasible as a Life Extension Strategy," *Medical Hypotheses* 72, no. 2 (February 2009): 125–28, doi: 10.1016/j.mehy.2008.07.044.

18. W. H. Tang et al., "Increased Trimethylamine N-Oxide Portends High Mortality Risk Independent of Glycemic Control in Patients with Type 2 Diabetes Mellitus,"*Clinical Chemistry* 63, no. 1 (January 2017): 297–306, doi: 10.1373/clinchem.2016.263640.

19. Stefan A. Ljunggren et al., "Persistent Organic Pollutants Distribution in Lipoprotein Fractions in Relation to Cardiovascular Disease and Cancer,"*Environment International* 65 (April 2014): 93–99, doi: 10.1016 /j.envint.2013.12.017.

20. L. Jiao et al., "Dietary Consumption of Meat, Fat, Animal Products and Advanced Glycation End-Products and the Risk of Barrett's Oesophagus,"*Alimentary Pharmacology & Therapeutics* 38, no. 7 (October 2013): 817–24, doi: 10.1111/apt.12459.

21. David Spero, "Do You Know Your Insulin Level?" *Diabetes Self-Management* (blog), October 23, 2013, diabetesselfmanagement.com/blog /do-you-know-your-insulin-level/.

22. A. E. Bunner et al., "A Dietary Intervention for Chronic Diabetic Neuropathy Pain: A Randomized Controlled Pilot Study," *Nutrition & Diabetes* 5 (May 2015): e158, doi: 10.1038/nutd.2015.8.

23. Dean Ornish, "A Radical Alternative for Democrats and Republicans," *Huffington Post* (blog), August 29, 2012, updated October 29, 2012, huffingtonpost.com/dr-dean-ornish/health-care-costs-treat-cause-symptom -prevention_b_1833789.html.

24. Teresa T. Fung et al., "Low-Carbohydrate Diets and All-Cause and Cause-Specific Mortality: Two Cohort Studies," *Annals of Internal Medicine* 153, no. 5 (September 7, 2010): 289–98, doi: 10.7326/0003-4819-153-5-201009070-00003.

Chapter 4: Slim and Trim

1. "Adult Obesity in the United States," The State of Obesity website, last modified September 1, 2016, stateofobesity.org/adult-obesity/.

2. G. M. Turner-McGrievy, N. D. Barnard, and A. R. Scialli, "A Two-Year Randomized Weight Loss Trial Comparing a Vegan Diet to a More Moderate Low-Fat Diet," *Obesity* 15, no. 9 (September 2007): 2276–81, doi: 10.1038/oby.2007.270.

3. S. Mishra et al., "A Multicenter Randomized Controlled Trial of a Plant-Based Nutrition Program to Reduce Body Weight and Cardiovascular Risk in the Corporate Setting: The GEICO Study," *European Journal of Clinical Nutrition* 67, no. 7 (July 2013): 718–24, doi: 10.1038/ejcn.2013.92.

4. R. Y. Huang et al., "Vegetarian Diets and Weight Reduction: A Meta-Analysis of Randomized Controlled Trials," *Journal of General Internal Medicine* 31, no. 1 (January 2016): 109–16, doi: 10.1007/s11606-015-3390-7.

5. G. M. Turner-McGrievy et al., "Comparative Effectiveness of Plant-Based Diets for Weight Loss: A Randomized Controlled Trial of Five Different Diets," *Nutrition* 31, no. 2 (February 2015): 350–58, doi: 10.1016/j.nut.2014.09.002.

6. S. Tonstad et al., "Type of Vegetarian Diet, Body Weight, and Prevalence of Type 2 Diabetes," *Diabetes Care* 32, no. 5 (May 2009): 791–96, doi: 10.2337/dc08-1886.

7. Keith Ayoob, "Op-Ed: Penn Jillette's Weight Loss Wasn't Magic," *MedPage Today* (blog), May 12, 2015, medpagetoday.com/Blogs/EdibleRx/51487.

Chapter 5: High on Plants for Low Blood Pressure

1. "High Blood Pressure Facts," Centers for Disease Control and Prevention, last modified November 30, 2016, cdc.gov/bloodpressure/facts.htm.

2. M. H. Forouzanfar et al., "Global, Regional, and National Comparative Risk Assessment of 79 Behavioural, Environmental and Occupational, and Metabolic Risks or Clusters of Risks, 1990–2015: A Systematic Analysis for the Global Burden of Disease Study 2015," *The Lancet* 388, no. 10053 (October 2016): 1659–1724, doi: 10.1016/S0140-6736(16)31679-8.

3. G. Fraser et al., "Vegetarian Diets and Cardiovascular Risk Factors in Black Members of the Adventist Health Study-2," *Public Health Nutrition* 18, no. 3 (February 2015): 537–45, doi: 10.1017/S1368980014000263.

4. B. J. Pettersen et al., "Vegetarian Diets and Blood Pressure Among White Subjects: Results from the Adventist Health Study-2 (AHS-2)," *Public Health Nutrition* 15, no. 10 (October 2012): 1909–16, doi: 10.1017/S1368980011003454.

5. J. McDougall et al., "Effects of 7 Days on an Ad Libitum Low-Fat Vegan Diet: The McDougall Program Cohort," *Nutrition Journal* 13 (October 2014): 99, doi: 10.1186/1475-2891-13-99.

6. P. N. Appleby, G. K. Davey, and T. J. Key, "Hypertension and Blood Pressure Among Meat Eaters, Fish Eaters, Vegetarians and Vegans in EPIC-Oxford," *Public Health Nutrition* 5, no. 5 (October 2002): 645–54, doi: 10.1079/PHN2002332.

Chapter 6: Hello Plants, Goodbye Cholesterol

1. "2015–2020 Dietary Guidelines: Answers to Your Questions," United States Department of Agriculture, last modified January 7, 2016, choosemyplate.gov/2015-2020-dietary-guidelines-answers-your-questions.

2. D. J. Jenkins et al., "Effects of a Dietary Portfolio of Cholesterol-Lowering Foods vs Lovastatin on Serum Lipids and C-Reactive Protein," *Journal of the American Medical Association* 290, no. 4 (July 23, 2003): 502–10, doi: 10.1001/jama.290.4.502.

3. K. E. Bradbury et al., "Serum Concentrations of Cholesterol, Apolipoprotein A-I and Apolipoprotein B in a Total of 1694 Meat Eaters, Fish Eaters, Vegetarians and Vegans," *European Journal of Clinical Nutrition* 68, no. 2 (February 2014): 178–83, doi: 10.1038/ejcn.2013.248.

4. Mishra et al., "The GEICO Study," 718–24.

5. A. Kuchta et al., "Impact of Plant-Based Diet on Lipid Risk Factors for Atherosclerosis," *Cardiology Journal* 23, no. 2 (2016): 141–48, doi: 10.5603/CJ.a2016.0002.

6. A. Malhotra, "Saturated Fat Is Not the Major Issue," *British Medical Journal* 347 (October 2013): f6340, doi: 10.1136/bmj.f6340.

7. P. W. Siri-Tarino et al., "Saturated Fatty Acids and Risk of Coronary Heart Disease: Modulation by Replacement Nutrients," *Current Atherosclerosis Reports* 12, no. 6 (November 2010): 384–90, doi: 10.1007/s11883-010-0131-6; R. Estruch et al., "Primary Prevention of Cardiovascular Disease with a Mediterranean Diet, *New England Journal*

of Medicine 368, no. 14 (April 4, 2013): 1279–90, doi: 10.1056 /NEJMoa1200303.

8. Fung et al, "Low-Carbohydrate Diets," 289–98.

Chapter 7: Grow Plants Not Cancer Cells

1. "Cancer Statistics," National Cancer Institute, last modified March 27, 2017, cancer.gov/about-cancer/understanding/statistics.

2. Ibid.

3. Ibid.

4. Xu Jiaquan et al., "Mortality in the United States, 2015," NCHS Data Brief No. 267, December 2016, Centers for Disease Control and Prevention, cdc .gov/nchs/products/databriefs/db267.htm.

5. International Agency for Research on Cancer, "IARC Monographs Evaluate Consumption of Red Meat and Processed Meat," press release, October 26, 2015, iarc.fr/en/media-centre/pr/2015/pdfs/pr240_E.pdf.

6. Peter Whoriskey, "Hot Dogs, Bacon and Other Processed Meats Cause Cancer, World Health Organization Declares," *The Washington Post,* October 26, 2015, washingtonpost.com/news/wonk/wp/2015/10/26 /hot-dogs-bacon-and-other-processed-meats-cause-cancer-world-health -organization-declares.

7. T. A. Hastert and E. White, "Association Between Meeting the WCRF /AICR Cancer Prevention Recommendations and Colorectal Cancer Incidence: Results from the VITAL Cohort, *Cancer Causes & Control* 27, no. 11 (November 2016): 1347–59, doi: 10.1007/s10552-016-0814-6.

8. Ibid.

9. "Colorectal Facts & Figures," American Cancer Society, accessed 5/22/17, cancer.org/research/cancerfactsstatistics/colorectal-cancer-facts-figures.

10. D. Ornish et al., "Intensive Lifestyle Changes May Affect the Progression of Prostate Cancer, *Journal of Urology* 174, no. 3 (September 2005): 1065–69, doi: 10.1097/01.ju.0000169487.49018.73.

11. Y. Tantamango-Bartley et al., "Are Strict Vegetarians Protected Against Prostate Cancer?" *American Journal of Clinical Nutrition* 103, no. 1 (January 2016): 153–60, doi: 10.3945/ajcn.114.106450.

12. M. J. Orlich et al., "Vegetarian Dietary Patterns and the Risk of Colorectal Cancers," *JAMA Internal Medicine* 175, no. 5 (May 2015): 767–76, doi: 10.1001/jamainternmed.2015.59.

13. T. J. Key et al., "Cancer in British Vegetarians: Updated Analyses of 4998 Incident Cancers in a Cohort of 32,491 Meat Eaters, 8612 Fish Eaters, 18,298 Vegetarians, and 2246 Vegans," *American Journal of Clinical Nutrition* 100, no. S1 (July 2014): S378–S85, doi: 10.3945 /ajcn.113.071266.

14. Jane V. Higdon et al, "Cruciferous Vegetables and Human Cancer Risk: Epidemiologic Evidence and Mechanistic Basis," *Pharmacological Research* 55, no. 3 (March 2007): 224–36, doi: 10.1016/j.phrs.2007.01.009.

15. M. Dinu et al., "Vegetarian, Vegan Diets and Multiple Health Outcomes: A Systematic Review with Meta-Analysis of Observational Studies," *Critical Reviews in Food Science and Nutrition* 57, no. 17 (November 2017): 3640–49, doi: 10.1080/10408398.2016.1138447.

Chapter 8: Beans Not Butter for Better Brains

1. "The Swank Low-Fat Diet for the Treatment of MS," The Swank MS Foundation, accessed 5/22/17, swankmsdiet.org/the-diet.

2. Julie Stachowiak, "What Is the Swank Diet for Multiple Sclerosis?" *Verywell* (blog), updated November 27, 2017, verywell.com /basic-rules-of-the-swank-diet-for-multiple-sclerosis-2440476.

3. R. L. Swank and B. B. Dugan, "Effect of Low Saturated Fat Diet in Early and Late Cases of Multiple Sclerosis," *The Lancet* 336, no. 8706 (July 7, 1990): 37–39, doi: 10.1016/0140-6736(90)91533-G.

4. R. L. Swank and J. Goodwin, "Review of MS Patient Survival on a Swank Low Saturated Fat Diet," *Nutrition* 19, no. 2 (February 2003): 161–62, doi: 10.1016/S0899-9007(02)00851-1.

5. P. Riccio, "The Molecular Basis of Nutritional Intervention in Multiple Sclerosis: A Narrative Review," *Complementary Therapies in Medicine* 19, no. 4 (August 2011): 228–37, doi: 10.1016/j.ctim.2011.06.006.

6. M. A. Kadoch, "Is the Treatment of Multiple Sclerosis Headed in the Wrong Direction?" *The Canadian Journal of Neurological Sciences* 39, no. 3 (May 2012): 405, doi: 10.1017/S0317167100022241.

7. John McDougall, "Results of the Diet & Multiple Sclerosis Study," *The McDougall Newsletter*, July 31, 2014, drmcdougall.com/2014/07/31 /results-of-the-diet-multiple-sclerosis-study.

8. L. T. Le and J Sabaté, "Beyond Meatless, the Health Effects of Vegan Diets: Findings from the Adventist Cohorts," *Nutrients* 6, no. 6 (May 27, 2014): 2131–47, doi: 10.3390/nu6062131.

9. P. Giem, W. L. Beeson, and G. E. Fraser, "The Incidence of Dementia and Intake of Animal Products: Preliminary Findings from the Adventist Health Study," *Neuroepidemiology* 12, no. 1 (1993): 28–36, doi: 10.1159/000110296.

10. N. D. Barnard et al., "Dietary and Lifestyle Guidelines for the Prevention of Alzheimer's Disease," *Neurobiology of Aging* 35, no. S2 (September 2014): S74–78, doi: 10.1016/j.neurobiolaging.2014.03.033.

11. B. L. Beezhold and C. S. Johnston, "Restriction of Meat, Fish, and Poultry in Omnivores Improves Mood: A Pilot Randomized Controlled Trial," *Nutrition Journal* 11 (February 14, 2012): 9, doi: 10.1186/1475-2891-11-9.

12. S. P. Shah and J. E. Duda, "Dietary Modifications in Parkinson's Disease: A Neuroprotective Intervention?" *Medical Hypotheses* 85, no. 6 (December 2015): 1002–05, doi: 10.1016/j.mehy.2015.08.018.

13. R. D. Abbott et al., "Frequency of Bowel Movements and the Future Risk of Parkinson's Disease,"*Neurology* 57, no. 3 (August 14, 2001): 456–62, doi: 10.1212/WNL.57.3.456.

14. M. A. Sanjoaquin et al., "Nutrition and Lifestyle in Relation to Bowel Movement Frequency: A Cross-Sectional Study of 20630 Men and Women in EPIC-Oxford," *Public Health Nutrition* 7, no. 1 (February 2004): 77–83, doi: 10.1079/PHN2003522.

15. Shah and Duda, "Dietary Modifications in Parkinson's Disease," 1002–05.

Chapter 9: Grow Plants Not Autoimmune Diseases

1. B. He et al., "Resetting Microbiota by Lactobacillus Reuteri Inhibits T Reg Deficiency-Induced Autoimmunity via Adenosine A2A Receptors," *The Journal of Experimental Medicine* 214, no. 1 (January 2017): 107–23, doi: 10.1084/jem.20160961.

2. J. M. Lyte, N. K. Gabler, and J. H. Hollis, "Postprandial Serum Endotoxin in Healthy Humans Is Modulated by Dietary Fat in a Randomized, Controlled, Cross-Over Study," *Lipids in Health and Disease* 15, no. 1 (November 5, 2016): 186, doi: 10.1186/s12944-016-0357-6.

3. L. Oates et al., "Reduction in Urinary Organophosphate Pesticide Metabolites in Adults After a Week-Long Organic Diet," *Environmental Research* 132 (July 2014): 105–11, doi: 10.1016/j.envres.2014.03.021.

4. Jörgen Magnér et al., *Human Exposure to Pesticides from Food: A Pilot Study* (Stockholm, Sweden: Swedish Environmental Research Institute, 2015), coop.se/PageFiles/430210/Coop%20Ekoeffekten_Rapport_eng.pdf.

5. S. Tonstad et al., "Prevalence of Hyperthyroidism According to Type of Vegetarian Diet," *Public Health Nutrition* 18, no. 8 (June 2015): 1482–87, doi: 10.1017/S1368980014002183.

6. S. Tonstad et al., "Vegan Diets and Hypothyroidism," *Nutrients* 5, no. 11 (November 20, 2013): 4642–52, doi: 10.3390/nu5114642.

Chapter 10: Plant-Powered GI and Kidney Systems

1. P. Jantchou et al., "Animal Protein Intake and Risk of Inflammatory Bowel Disease: The E3N Prospective Study," *American Journal of Gastroenterology* 105, no. 10 (October 2010): 2195–201, doi: 10.1038/ajg.2010.192.

2. M. Chiba et al., "Lifestyle-Related Disease in Crohn's Disease: Relapse Prevention by a Semi-Vegetarian Diet," *World Journal of Gastroenterology* 16, no. 20 (May 28, 2010): 2484–95, doi: 10.3748/wjg.v16.i20.2484.

3. Y. Tantamango-Bartley et al., "Vegetarian Diets and the Incidence of Cancer in a Low-Risk Population," *Cancer Epidemiology Biomarkers & Prevention* 22, no. 2 (February 2013): 286–94, doi: 10.1158/1055-9965.EPI-12-1060.

4. F. L. Crowe et al., "Diet and Risk of Diverticular Disease in Oxford Cohort of European Prospective Investigation into Cancer and Nutrition (EPIC): Prospective Study of British Vegetarians and Non-Vegetarians," *British Medical Journal* 343 (July 19, 2011): d4131, doi: 10.1136/bmj.d4131.

5. V. Wiwanitkit, "Renal Function Parameters of Thai Vegans Compared with Non-Vegans," *Renal Failure* 29, no. 2 (2007): 219–20, doi: 10.1080/08860220601098912.

6. J. Lin, F. B. Hu, and G. C. Curhan, "Associations of Diet with Albuminuria and Kidney Function Decline," *Clinical Journal of the American Society of Nephrology* 5, no. 5 (May 2010): 836–43, doi: 10.2215/CJN.08001109.

7. Ibid.

8. S. M. Moe et al., "Vegetarian Compared with Meat Dietary Protein Source and Phosphorus Homeostasis in Chronic Kidney Disease," *Clinical Journal of the American Society of Nephrology* 6, no. 2 (February 2011): 257–64, doi: 10.2215/CJN.05040610.

9. B. W. Turney et al., "Diet and Risk of Kidney Stones in the Oxford Cohort of the European Prospective Investigation into Cancer and Nutrition (EPIC)," *European Journal of Epidemiology* 29, no. 5 (May 2014): 363–69, doi: 10.1007/s10654-014-9904-5.

Chapter 11: Fifty Shades of Green with Plants and Sex

1. "FOK Releases 'Raise the Flag with a Vegan Diet' about Sexual Dysfunction," *Forks Over Knives* (blog), January 24, 2012, forksoverknives.com /fok-releases-raising-the-flag-with-a-vegan-diet-about-sexual-dysfunction.

2. Bolaji Oyetunde Oyelade et al., "Prevalence of Erectile Dysfunction and Possible Risk Factors Among Men of South-Western Nigeria: A Population Based Study," *The Pan African Medical Journal* 24 (2016): 124, doi: 10.11604/pamj.2016.24.124.8660.

3. A. Cassidy, M. Franz, and E. B. Rimm, "Dietary Flavonoid Intake and Incidence of Erectile Dysfunction," *American Journal of Clinical Nutrition* 103, no. 2 (February 2016): 534–41, doi: 10.3945/ajcn.115.122010.

4. K. Esposito et al., "Mediterranean Diet Improves Erectile Function in Subjects with the Metabolic Syndrome," *International Journal of Impotence Research* 18, no. 4 (July–August 2006): 405–10, doi: 10.1038 /sj.ijir.3901447.

Chapter 12: The Garden of Youth

1. D. Ornish et al., "Increased Telomerase Activity and Comprehensive Lifestyle Changes: A Pilot Study," *The Lancet Oncology* 9, no. 11 (November 2008): 1048–57, doi: 10.1016/S1470-2045(08)70234-1.

2. D. Ornish et al., "Changes in Prostate Gene Expression in Men Undergoing an Intensive Nutrition and Lifestyle Intervention," *Proceedings of the National Academy of Sciences of the United States of America* 105, no. 24 (June 17, 2008): 8369–74, doi: 10.1073/pnas.0803080105.

3. D. L. Ellsworth et al., "Intensive Cardiovascular Risk Reduction Induces Sustainable Changes in Expression of Genes and Pathways Important to Vascular Function," *Circulation: Cardiovascular Genetics* 7, no. 2 (April 2014): 151–60, doi: 10.1161/CIRCGENETICS.113.000121.

4. J. A. Monro, R. Leon, and B. K. Puri, "The Risk of Lead Contamination in Bone Broth Diets," *Medical Hypotheses* 80, no. 4 (April 2013): 389–90, doi: 10.1016/j.mehy.2012.12.026.

5. J. Cha, A. Niedzwiecki, and M. Rath, "Hypoascorbemia Induces Atherosclerosis and Vascular Deposition of Lipoprotein(A) in Transgenic Mice," *American Journal of Cardiovascular Disease* 5, no. 1 (March 20, 2015): 53–62, ncbi.nlm.nih.gov/pubmed/26064792.

6. O. Castañer et al., "In Vivo Transcriptomic Profile After a Mediterranean Diet in High-Cardiovascular Risk Patients: A Randomized Controlled Trial,"

American Journal of Clinical Nutrition 98, no. 3 (September 2013): 845–53, doi: 10.3945/ajcn.113.060582.

Chapter 13: Plants, the Plight of Animals, and World Religions

1. "Factory Farming: The Truth Behind the Barn Doors," *Last Chance for Animals*, accessed 5/22/17, lcanimal.org/index.php/campaigns/other-issues /factory-farming.

2. Carrie Hribar, *Understanding Concentrated Animal Feeding Operations and Their Impact on Communities*, ed. Mark Schultz (Bowling Green, Ohio: National Association of Local Boards of Health, 2010), cdc.gov/nceh/ehs /docs/understanding_cafos_nalboh.pdf.

3. "The Best Speech You Will Ever Hear—Gary Yourofsky," YouTube video, 1:10:22, from a speech made at Georgia Tech in 2010, posted by "TheAnimalHolocaust," December 22, 2010, youtube.com /watch?v=es6U00LMmC4&sns=fb.

4. Adaptt: Animals Deserve Absolute Protection Today and Tomorrow, website of Gary Yourofsky, adaptt.org.

5. C. Radnitz, B. Beezhold, and J. DiMatteo, "Investigation of Lifestyle Choices of Individuals Following a Vegan Diet for Health and Ethical Reasons," *Appetite* 90 (July 2015): 31–36, doi: 10.1016/j .appet.2015.02.026.

6. Human Rights Code, R.S.O., chapter H.19 (1990) (Ontario, Can.), ontario.ca/laws/statute/90h19.

7. Ibid.

8. Ibid.

9. The Daniel Plan, website of the lifestyle program of the same name, danielplan.com.

10. "Living a Healthful Life," Seventh-day Adventist Church website, accessed 5/22/17, adventist.org/en/vitality/health.

11. Jesus People for Animals, PETA, jesuspeopleforanimals.com or petalambs.com.

12. Richard C. Foltz, "Is Vegetarianism Un-Islamic?" *Studies in Contemporary Islam* 3, no. 1 (2001): 39–54, reposted on Animals in Islam, PETA, animalsinislam.com/islam-animal-rights/vegetarianism-un-islamic.

13. Shabkar, website dedicated to vegetarianism for Buddhists, last modified March 17, 2017, shabkar.org.

14. "Jainism," Hinduwebsite.com, accessed 5/22/17, hinduwebsite.com /jainism/jainindex.asp.

15. "North America: Early 20th Century/Albert Einstein (1879–1955)," International Vegetarian Union, accessed 5/22/17, ivu.org/history /northam20a/einstein.html.

16. "Sir Paul McCartney Narrates 'Glass Walls,'" Action Centre page, PETA UK, accessed 5/22/17, action.peta.org.uk/ea-action/action?ea.client .id=5&ea.campaign.id=5133.

Chapter 14: The Earthen Plate and the Environment

1. "The Disappearing Rainforests," Save the Amazon Coalition website, accessed 5/22/17, savetheamazon.org/rainforeststats.htm.

2. Ibid.

3. Julia Loman, "Medicinal Secrets of the Amazon Rainforest," *Julia's Journal* (blog), Amazon Aid Foundation, March 31, 2016, amazonaid.org /medicinal-secrets-of-the-amazon.

4. "Amazon Rainforest," Greenpeace USA, accessed 5/22/17, greenpeace.org /usa/forests/amazon-rainforest.

5. "Cattle Ranching in the Amazon Region," Global Forest Atlas, Yale School of Forestry and Environmental Studies, accessed 5/22/17, globalforestatlas .yale.edu/amazon/land-use/cattle-ranching.

6. Jon Dettling et al., *A Comparative Life Cycle Assessment of Plant-Based Foods and Meat Foods* (Boston, MA: Quantis USA, 2016), prepared for MorningStar Farms, accessed 5/22/17, morningstarfarms.com/content/dam /morningstarfarms/pdf/MSFPlantBasedLCAReport_2016-04-10_Final.pdf.

7. John Gaudiosi, "James Cameron: Why I Eat a Vegan Diet," interview with James Cameron, *Men's Journal*, accessed 5/22/17, mensjournal.com /health-fitness/nutrition/james-cameron-why-i-eat-a-vegan-diet-20150915.

8. Ibid.

9. Marco Springmann et al., "Analysis and Valuation of the Health and Climate Change Cobenefits of Dietary Change," *Proceedings of the National Academy of Sciences of the United States* 113, no. 15 (March 21, 2016): 4146–51, doi: 10.1073/pnas.1523119113.

10. E. Hertwich et al., United Nations Environment Programme, *Assessing the Environmental Impacts of Consumption and Production: Priority Products and Materials*, A Report of the Working Group on the Environmental Impacts of Products and Materials to the International Panel for Sustainable

Resource Management (Paris, France: UNEP, 2010), accessed 5/22/17, unep.fr/shared/publications/pdf/DTIx1262xPA -PriorityProductsAndMaterials_Report.pdf.

11. Naomi Imatome-Yun, "Federal Report Finds Plant-Based Diet Is Best; Meat Industry Is Unhappy," *Forks Over Knives* (blog), April 6, 2015, forksoverknives .com/federal-report-finds-plant-based-diet-is-best-meat-industry-is-unhappy/.

12. "Scientific Report of the 2015 Dietary Guidelines Advisory Committee," Office of Disease Prevention and Health Promotion, health.gov /dietaryguidelines/2015-scientific-report/10-chapter-5/d5-3.asp.

13. T. J. Vilsack and S. M. M. Burwell, "2015 Dietary Guidelines: Giving You the Tools You Need to Make Healthy Choices," US Department of Agriculture blog, October 6, 2015, blogs.usda.gov/2015/10/06/2015 -dietary-guidelines-giving-you-the-tools-you-need-to-make-healthy-choices.

14. S. B. Eaton and M. Konner, "Paleolithic Nutrition: A Consideration of Its Nature and Current Implications," *New England Journal of Medicine* 312, no. 5 (January 31, 1985): 283–89, doi: 10.1056/NEJM198501313120505.

15. P. Scarborough et al., "Dietary Greenhouse Gas Emissions of Meat -Eaters, Fish-Eaters, Vegetarians and Vegans in the UK," *Climate Change* 125, no. 2 (2014): 179–92, doi: 10.1007/s10584-014-1169-1; Gidon Eshel et al., "Environmentally Optimal, Nutritionally Aware Beef Replacement Plant-Based Diets," *Environmental Science and Technology* 50, no. 15 (2016): 8164–68, doi: 10.1021/acs.est.6b01006.

16. "Is a Vegetarian Paleo Diet Possible—S. Boyd Eaton," YouTube video, 0:35, from a statement made at Finding Common Ground conference on November 17, 2015, posted by "Oldways," January 19, 2016, youtube .com/watch?v=Qx9OfvjedhM.

Resources

My goal has been to be thorough but not exhaustive in the content and references in this book. There are so many web-based resources that I rely on, ones I recommend you be familiar with too. They contain a wealth of information that no single book could ever contain. Here are some of the most useful.

Science Resources

US National Library of Medicine, pubmed.com. This site comprises millions of PubMed articles going back over 100 years. Only some are available in their full content. I usually search for these preferentially and might limit my search to human studies. For example, searching vegetarian diets today there are 3,173 scientific entries. For the Paleo diet, there are 142.

Physicians Committee for Responsible Medicine, pcrm.org. You have read about many of the studies done by Dr. Neal Barnard and colleagues from this organization. There is a section on cancer and diet that is superb. There are many recipes as a bonus.

NutritionFacts.org, nutritionfacts.org. Signing up for the daily video and email blasts on science related to nutrition should be mandatory for everyone in the health field, which is everyone.

ScienceDaily, sciencedaily.com. This site is a way to keep up to date on new science distilled down to digestible chunks. It is not necessarily a vegan site.

Environmental Working Group, ewg.org. The EWG provides in-depth information on toxins in food and personal-use items.

Animal Rights Resources

People for the Ethical Treatment of Animals, peta.org. This is a great site for increasing your knowledge and commitment to animal rights.

Animals Deserve Absolute Protection Today and Tomorrow, adaptt.org. This site by Gary Yourofsky is the real deal for animal liberation.

Mercy for Animals, mercyforanimals.org. This is an animal advocacy organization that does an amazing job of education and programming for all ages.

Farm Sanctuary, farmsanctuary.org. This organization rescues abused animals and educates on the plight of animals. With several locations across the United States, it has done an amazing job in the past thirty years.

Recipes and Guides Resources

VegSource, vegsource.com. This site has many recipes and informative articles.

The Plant-Based Dietitian, plantbaseddietitian.com. This is the work of all-star dietitian Julieanna Hever from LA. Her videos, recipes, and articles are amazing.

Plant Based Nutrition Support Group, pbnsg.org. This site provides amazing recipes and articles.

Ornish Lifestyle Medicine, ornish.com. This is the site for Dr. Dean Ornish. It is rich in articles and recipes.

Dr. Esselstyn's Prevent & Reverse Heart Disease Program, dresselstyn.com. This is the site for Dr. Caldwell Esselstyn and is a great place for articles, videos, and recipes.

Dr. McDougall's Health & Medical Center, drmcdougall.com. This is the site for Dr. John McDougall. His starch-based recipes and his pithy articles are not to be missed.

Forks Over Knives, forksoverknives.com. This is the site for the documentary by the same name and the recipes and cookbooks that have helped so many succeed at WFPB diets.

VegNews, vegnews.com. This is a widely read magazine, online and in print, that has news and recipes to keep up to date on the latest trends.

Residential Programs Resources

Hippocrates Health Institute, hippocratesinst.org. This is the predominantly raw WFPB treatment center in West Palm Beach, Florida, that has been a haven and healing site to many.

Pritikin Longevity Center + Spa, pritikin.com. This site has so many resources that you will want to visit the Miami resort.

TrueNorth Health Center, healthpromoting.com. This is the site for the TrueNorth Health Center in California. For over twenty years this plant-based center has used diet and fasting to heal many people.

Tree of Life Center US, treeoflifecenterus.com. This is where Dr. Gabriel Cousens has been using raw diets and spiritual paths to heal patients from around the world. It is in the desert outside of Tucson, Arizona.

Restaurants

GreenSpace Café, greenspacecafe.com. This is the site for my restaurant in Ferndale, Michigan. It is one of the finest WFPB eateries anywhere.

List of Recipes

Index

About the Author

D r. Joel K. Kahn is America's Healthy Heart Doc after serving in that role for *Reader's Digest Magazine*. He is a summa cum laude graduate of the University of Michigan School of Medicine and has been certified in internal medicine, cardiovascular medicine, interventional cardiology, nuclear cardiology, and metabolic medicine. He is the founder of the Kahn Center for Cardiac Longevity in Bloomfield Hills, Michigan, and has opened several popular health-food restaurants. Dr. Kahn has published over 100 scientific articles on heart disease and many book chapters in textbooks. He serves as a clinical professor of medicine at Wayne State University School of Medicine. He is a regular contributor to the *Huffington Post* and other outlets and is a health consultant to Fox 2 Detroit. He has a public TV special on heart disease that has played nationally. He received a Health Care Hero award in 2016 from *Crain's Detroit Business* and was named the Sexiest Male Vegan Over 50 by PETA in 2016.

About Sounds True

Sounds True is a multimedia publisher whose mission is to inspire and support personal transformation and spiritual awakening. Founded in 1985 and located in Boulder, Colorado, we work with many of the leading spiritual teachers, thinkers, healers, and visionary artists of our time. We strive with every title to preserve the essential "living wisdom" of the author or artist. It is our goal to create products that not only provide information to a reader or listener but also embody the quality of a wisdom transmission.

For those seeking genuine transformation, Sounds True is your trusted partner. At SoundsTrue.com you will find a wealth of free resources to support your journey, including exclusive weekly audio interviews, free downloads, interactive learning tools, and other special savings on all our titles.

To learn more, please visit SoundsTrue.com/freegifts or call us toll-free at 800.333.9185.

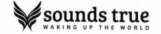